KETO COPYCAT

85 TASTY, HEALTHY, AND EASY RECIPES TO PREPARE YOUR FAVORITE RESTAURANT DISHES AT HOME WHILE ON A KETO DIET

Table of Contents

INTRODUCTION
- What Is Ketogenic Diet?
- What Can I Eat on a Ketogenic Diet?
- What Foods Should I Avoid?
- Benefits of Keto Diet
- What Are Copycat Recipes?
- Why Copycat Recipes?

CHAPTER 1: BREAKFAST KETO RECIPES
1. Starbucks Walnut Banana Bread
2. Doctor Seuss Green Eggs and Hams
3. Tim Hortons Iced Capps
4. The Pancake Princess Rhubarb Coconut Pancake
5. Starbucks Egg Muffins with Steak Strips
6. Starbucks Pumpkin Bread
7. International House of Pancakes' Fluffy Coconut Pancakes
8. Pat's King Bacon and Egg Breakfast Wraps with Salsa and Avocado
9. McGriddle Bacon Sandwiches
10. Kind Bars

CHAPTER 2: LUNCH KETO RECIPES
11. Longhorn's Parmesan Crusted Chicken
12. Panda Express Kung Pao Chicken
13. Chang's Lettuce Wraps
14. Asian Chicken Taco Lettuce Wraps
15. KFC Fried Chicken
16. Tso's Shrimp and Broccoli
17. Long John Silver's Batter-Dipped Fish
18. Olive Garden's Steak Gorgonzola Alfredo
19. Chipotle's Chipotle Pork Carnitas
20. Red Lobster's Shrimp Scampi with Cheddar Bay Biscuits
21. Outback Steakhouse Charcoal Ribeye
22. Chicken Pan with Veggies and Pesto
23. Creamy Garlic Chicken
24. Chinese Pork Bowl
25. Turkey-Pepper Mix
26. Simple Tuna Salad
27. Chipotle Steak with Tortilla

28. Bacon-Wrapped Chicken Breast
29. Spinach Stuffed Salmon
30. Creamy Zoodles

CHAPTER 3: DINNER KETO RECIPES

31. Creamy Chicken and Mushroom Casserole
32. Skillet Chicken Florentine
33. Turkey Casserole
34. Turkey with Cream-Cheese Sauce
35. Steak Cobb Salad with Cilantro Lime Vinaigrette
36. Crispy Sesame Beef
37. Fat Bomb Pork Chops
38. Italian Sausage Stuffed Mushrooms
39. Lamb Chops with Herb Butter
40. Lamb Burgers
41. Fish in Lemon Butter Caper Sauce
42. Creamy Garlic Shrimp
43. Spicy Almond Tofu
44. Vegan Dinner Bowl
45. Cheese Quiche Stuffed Peppers

CHAPTER 4: VEGAN KETO RECIPES

46. P. F. Chang's® Spicy Green Beans
47. Applebee® Veggie Patch Pizza
48. Applebee® Vegetable Medley
49. PF Chang's® Shanghai Cucumbers
50. Chili® Black Bean
51. In "N" Out® Animal Style Fries
52. KFC® Coleslaw
53. Cracker Barrel® Baby Carrot
54. Olive Garden® Gnocchi with Spicy Tomato and Wine Sauce
55. Chipotle® Sofritas
56. Melting Pot® Green Goddess Dip
57. Applebee's Onion Peels
58. McDonald's® Hash Browns
59. P. F. Chang's® Vegetarian Lettuce Wraps
60. Houston® Veggie Burger
61. Disneyland® Chili Lime Corn on the Cob
62. Tony Roma® Maple Sweet Potatoes
63. Ruby Tuesday® Creamy Mashed Cauliflower
64. P. F. Chang's® Garlic Snap Peas
65. Lone Star Steakhouse & Saloon® Baked Sweet Potato

CHAPTER 5: SPECIAL OCCASION KETO RECIPES

66. Taquitos
67. Zucchini Tater Tots
68. Bell Pepper Nachos
69. Buffalo Style Shrimp in Lettuce Wraps
70. Baby Back Ribs
71. Grilled Buffalo Wings
72. Brie & Caramelized Onion Burgers
73. Chicken Zoodle Casserole
74. Spicy Tuna Stuffed Avocados
75. Pesto Salmon

CHAPTER 6: DESSERT KETO RECIPES

76. Strawberry Shortcake (The Cheesecake Factory)
77. Chocolate Glazed Donuts (Dunkin Donuts)
78. Muffins (Dunkin Donuts)
79. Frosted Fudge Brownies (Panera Bread)
80. Cinnamon Scones (Panera)

CONCLUSION

Introduction

What Is Ketogenic Diet?

The ketogenic diet is a low-carb, moderate-protein and high-fat diet. It forces your body into a state where it switches from using glucose for fuel to ketones. Ketones are created in the liver and fatty acids are used as energy when blood sugar (glucose) is not available to the cells. Glucose comes from carbohydrates like bread, pasta, rice or fructose from fruit!

What Can I Eat on a Ketogenic Diet?

Eating keto means eating foods that have high fat content with moderate protein and very limited carbs. Carbs are the enemy! Strictly limit your carbohydrate intake to 20–30g per day. In case you are an athlete, you may need to go up to 50g per day. However, this isn't necessary for weight loss. The ketogenic diet focuses on the major sources of carbs—bread, pastas and rice—and eliminates them completely.

What Foods Should I Avoid?

In ketogenic diet, you need to avoid foods which are high in carbohydrates. They are:

- All Grains (Wheat, Corn, Rice, Rye, etc.)
- Sugar and Sweeteners (Agave Nectar, Honey, Maple Syrup)
- Excessive Fruit (Berries) and Non-Starchy Vegetables (Broccoli)
- Legumes — Beans or Peas like Lentils or Peanuts.

The following foods should be eaten only occasionally or in small portions when needed:

- White Potato — Cooked or Raw — Avoid completely unless it is your only choice. In this case go for a maximum of 4 oz per day.
- Abstain from artificial sweeteners like: Aspartame, Equal, NutraSweet, Splenda.

- Remember that soda and fruit juices are not considered as a keto food. They are high in sugar and won't help you to lose weight!

Benefits of Keto Diet

There is a long list of Ketogenic Diet Benefits. Following are few:

- It promotes weight loss and inhibits hunger.
- The diet relieves you from various health conditions such as type 2 diabetes, epilepsy, Alzheimer's disease, Parkinson's disease and cancer.
- It gives your body a complete rest by providing the essential nutrients the body needs.
- Increased energy levels due to the intake of healthy fats.
- You will be able to control your blood sugar levels, improve cholesterol and decrease your risk for heart disease.

This book is not only about keto diet but also copycat recipes, let us proceed.

What Are Copycat Recipes?

Copycat Recipes are based on at-home versions of the most popular restaurant meals. Some of our favorite foods, from around the world, are in this book.

Why Copycat Recipes?

We all love to eat out. When we go to a restaurant, we want variety and quality. Restaurant meals allow us to eat out without having to be creative or cook for ourselves.

It's so much more fun and cost effective to recreate restaurant style recipes yourself.

There's another benefit of cooking copycat recipe, it will save you lots of money! You can learn how much the cost is for each ingredient in your favorite dishes, then substitute with less expensive alternatives when you cook at home!

Keto copycat recipes are very popular. These are recipes that are based on food items from popular restaurants. These recipes are great for keto diet, since they are low in carbohydrates and high in fats. The book will allow you to make copycat versions of your favorite restaurant meals at home.

This book aims to give readers simple recipes that will help you replicate your favorite restaurant meals in your home and for people who don't enjoy a lot of cooking or have no time for it. We have carefully curated the recipes and we believe that they are easy to make and will be an excellent choice for your family dinners.

Chapter 1: Breakfast Keto Recipes

1. Starbucks Walnut Banana Bread

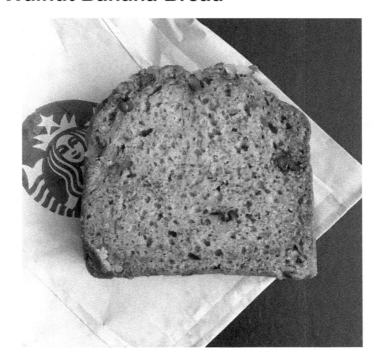

Preparation Time: 5 Minutes

Cooking Time: 25 Minutes

Servings: 4

Ingredients:

- 1 cup of almond flour (alternative: flaxseed)
- 1/2 cup of coconut flour
- 1/2 cup of coconut oil melted

- 2 tsp. of ground cinnamon
- 1/2 cup of golden flax meal
- 3/4 cup Sukrin Gold/substitution sugar
- 2 tsp. of maple syrup sugar-free
- 5–6 drops of banana extract
- 1 tbsp. of vanilla extract
- 2 tbsp. of psyllium powder
- 1/4 tbsp. of nutmeg
- 1/4 tbsp. of sea salt
- 3 tsp. of baking powder
- 3/4 cups of chopped walnuts
- 4 large eggs
- 1/2 cup of almond or coconut milk

Directions:

1. Preheat oven to 350ºF.
2. Grease, and then cover a 9x5 loaf pan with parchment paper.
3. Mix the dry ingredients in a medium-sized bowl: almond flour, coconut meal, sea salt, baking powder, psyllium powder, flax meal, and spices.
4. Melt the coconut oil, and then allow it to cool.
5. Add the coconut oil with the substitute sugar, maple syrup, banana extract, and vanilla.
6. Then beat the eggs one by one.

7. Adding the combined dry ingredients to the wet batter, beat until fully absorbed at a low-medium level.

8. Add the almond or coconut milk half cup, then start stirring.

9. Next mix in the walnuts, reserving a few tbsp. to add the banana loaf to the top right before baking.

10. Place the batter in a well-grained 9X5 loaf pan and cover it with parchment paper.

11. Bake for 35–40 minutes at 350ºF or until a toothpick of the inserted comes out clean.

12. Leave the bread to cool completely before slicing.

13. Keep in the refrigerator until 5 days or freeze for up to 3 weeks.

Nutrition:

- Calories: 400
- Proteins: 9g
- Carbs: 10g
- Fat: 23g
- Fiber: 0g

2. Doctor Seuss Green Eggs and Hams

Preparation Time: 5 Minutes

Cooking Time: 15 Minutes

Servings: 1

Ingredients:

- 1/8 cup of Parmesan cheese
- 3 tsp. of nuts
- 5 pieces of fresh garlic cloves
- 2 tbsp. of parsley
- 1 tbsp. of basil
- 3/4 cup of olive oil extra virgin
- Citrus juice/lime juice
- Season with sea salt
- 2 eggs
- 1 tbsp. of heavy cream
- 1 tbsp. of butter
- 1 tbsp. of keto basil pesto
- ¼ cup of ham
- ¼ cup of mushrooms

- 1 tbsp. of butter
- 1 tbsp. of cheese
- Pinch of paprika
- Dry oregano
- Red flakes chilly
- Black pepper and sea salt

Directions:

1. Grate the Parmesan cheese and blend with the garlic and pine nuts
2. Pair with spinach, olive oil, lemon juice, and sea salt
3. Blend into a smooth paste. Keep in the refrigerator, using in pasta or even on pizza
4. Mix the eggs with the whipping cream and pesto, and beat it.
5. Heat the butter in a pan.
6. Turn the heat down to the lowest and pour in the eggs.
7. Keep scrambling the eggs around in the pan and let them cook slow and steady.
8. Once done, remove and serve.
9. Heat the butter in a pan.
10. Add in the paprika, oregano, and chili flakes.
11. Fry the ham and cook until crisp to your liking.
12. In the same pan, add the mushrooms.
13. Season with sea salt and black pepper.
14. Grate some cheese over the mushrooms.

15.   Once the cheese has melted, remove, and serve.

Nutrition:

- Calories: 160
- Proteins: 20g
- Carbs: 2g
- Fat: 10g
- Fiber: 2g

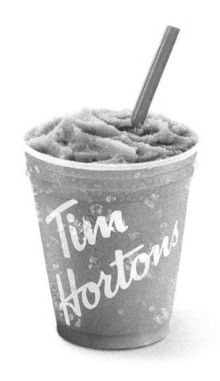

3. Tim Hortons Iced Capps

Preparation Time: 3 Minutes

Cooking Time: 10 Minutes

Servings: 2

Ingredients:

- 4 cups of ice cubes
- 2 cups of prepared coffee

- 1/2 tsp. vanilla
- 1/3 cup of heavy whipping cream
- 4 tbsp. erythritol (or favorite sweetener)

Directions:

1. Make two cups of your favorite coffee.
2. Mix all the ingredients in a mixer, ice, cream, vanilla, erythritol, and coffee.
3. Pulse it 4,5 times till completely mixed together.
4. Pour in mugs.

Nutrition:

- Calories: 232
- Proteins: 6g
- Carbs: 20g
- Fat: 8g
- Fiber: 0g

4. The Pancake Princess Rhubarb Coconut Pancake

Preparation Time: 5 Minutes

Cooking Time: 15 Minutes

Servings: 6

Ingredients:

- 2 tbsp. olive oil
- 1/4 cup of coconut flour
- 2 tbsp. of maple syrup (sugar-free)
- 1 tsp. of baking powder
- 3 large eggs
- 1 tsp. of vanilla extract
- 1 cup of rhubarb (make a fine paste)
- 1/8 tsp. of fine sea salt

Directions:

1. Combine the eggs, maple syrup, coconut flour, vanilla extract, oil, baking powder, and sea salt in a big bowl. Use a hand beater to mix it, so there will not be any clumps left.

2. Add three tbsp. of the pancake batter in a buttered skillet on medium-low heat; let it cook until bubbles arise in the pancake for about 4 to 5 minutes.

3. After it has cooked from one side, turn the pancake on the other side and let it cook on the other side for about 4 minutes, or until both sides are brown. Do not increase the heat to speed up the cooking time, or the pancake's outsides will burn before the inside is cooked completely.

4. Repeat the process with the leftover batter; it will make roughly six small pancakes. Remaining pancake batter can be stored in an airtight jar in the cool place or fridge for almost 3 days.

Nutrition:

- Calories: 400
- Proteins: 20g
- Carbs: 20g
- Fat: 10g
- Fiber: 2g

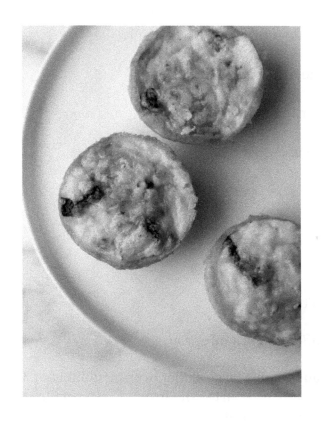

5. Starbucks Egg Muffins with Steak Strips

Preparation Time: 10 Minutes

Cooking Time: 15 Minutes

Servings: 12

Ingredients:

- 1/4 cup of chopped bell black peppers
- 3/4 cup of sausage

- 1/2 cup of spinach (frozen)
- 8 large eggs
- 1/4 cup of heavy cream
- 1 cup shredded of cheddar cheese
- 1/4 tsp. of garlic powder
- Sea salt: to taste
- 1/2 tsp. of black pepper
- Steak strips (your choice)

Directions:

1. Preheat oven to 350ºF.
2. Spray the muffin tin with oil spray.
3. Brown the sausage in a large skillet over medium heat. Using a spatula or wooden spoon to split the link apart while it cooks into smaller parts. Move the sausage to a small bowl, and then put aside to cool.
4. Sauté the spinach and black peppers in a wide skillet until the vegetables are soft, around 5 minutes. Remove from heat, and then put aside to cool.
5. Whisk together heavy cream, the eggs, and 3/4 cup of shredded cheese in a medium-size mixing bowl. Mix with the garlic powder, sea salt, and black pepper. Add the sausage and vegetables cooked in. Combine well.
6. Uniformly distribute the batter into the muffin pan. Sprinkle with the remaining 1/4 cup of melted cheese over the muffins.
7. Bake for around 18–20 minutes or until the eggs are completely done.

Nutrition:

- Calories: 300

- Proteins: 40g
- Carbs: 20g
- Fat: 20g

6. Starbucks Pumpkin Bread

Preparation Time: 10 Minutes

Cooking Time: 50 Minutes

Servings: 6

Ingredients:

- 4 large eggs
- 1/2 cup of butter, softened
- 3/4 cup of pumpkin puree
- 1 tsp. of vanilla extract
- 2/3 cup of erythritol sweetener
- 1 1/2 cup of almond flour (alternative: flaxseed)
- 4 tsp. of baking powder
- 1 tsp. of cinnamon
- 1/2 tsp. of nutmeg
- 1/2 cup of coconut flour
- 1/4 tsp. of ginger
- 1/8 tsp. of cloves
- 1/2 tsp. of sea salt

Directions:

1. Turn on the oven for it to preheat to 350ºF. Grease a 9x5" loaf pan and line with butter paper.

2. In a big mixing bowl, add the sweetener, butter, and together mix until light and airy.

3. One by one, add the eggs and mix.

4. Then add the vanilla extract, pumpkin puree, and mix it well.

5. Stir together the almond flour, coconut flour, baking powder, cinnamon, nutmeg, ginger, cloves, and sea salt in a different bowl. Whisk it well.

6. Now combine wet and dry ingredients.

7. Optionally, add up to 1/2 cup of mix-ins, like chopped nuts or chocolate chips. The batter will be thick and sticky.

8. Take the prepared loaf pan and pour batter into it. Bake for 45–55 minutes.

9. If the bread is browning too quickly, you can cover the pan with a piece of aluminum foil.

10. Enjoy!

Nutrition:

- Calories: 235
- Proteins: 4g
- Carbs: 26g
- Fat: 2g
- Fiber: 2g

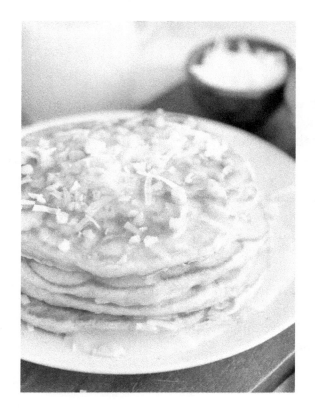

7. International House of Pancakes' Fluffy Coconut Pancakes

Preparation Time: 5 Minutes

Cooking Time: 25 Minutes

Servings: 12

Ingredients:

- 3 eggs(add another egg if the batter becomes too thick)
- 1/4 cup of melted use salted butter or sea-salted

- 1/4 cup of heavy crème or sour crème
- 1 Stevia Packet
- 1/4 tsp. of sea salt
- 1/2 tsp. of vanilla extract
- 1/4 cup of coconut flour
- 1/2 tsp. of baking powder

Directions:

1. Mix stevia, butter, eggs, cream, and sea salt, with vanilla extract.
2. Combine coconut flour with baking powder.
3. Combine dry ingredients and wet ingredients.
4. Thicken the batter by letting it sit.
5. Spray the skillet with oil spray and heat on medium heat.
6. Pour tbsp. of batter onto skillet to make pancakes about two-3 inches in diameter.
7. Make the pancake flat by spoon because the batter is too thick.
8. The initial recipe called 4 whites, but practice proved 3 were stronger and less eggy for the pancakes. You should use only the whites with 2 of the yolks, with an even less eggy flavor. When the batter is so dense, extra cream may be used so.
9. This batter makes 12 pancakes consisting of small size coconut flour. Unless the scale is larger than 2–3 inches long, you can get fewer. Nutritional evidence is based on 2 pancakes per serving, which means 12.
10. The batter is meant to be dense and should thicken as it lies. As it is a thick batter, it can be spread out a little with a spoon if desired after putting on the griddle.
11. When the exterior is browning up until the inside starts cooking, the cooking temperature would be too high. Check with a tiny single pancake to ensure the

temperature is correct before introducing more. It is also a successful method for making changes to the batter before preparing the entire pan, if appropriate.

Nutrition:

- Calories: 340
- Proteins: 20g
- Carbs: 30g
- Fat: 20g
- Fiber: 3g

8. Pat's King Bacon and Egg Breakfast Wraps with Salsa and Avocado

Preparation Time: 5 Minutes

Cooking Time: 15 Minutes

Servings: 4

Ingredients:

- 2 large eggs
- 2 pieces of low-carb wraps
- 3 slices of bacon
- Sea salt and black pepper (to taste)
- 1/2 cup of grated cheddar cheese
- 1/2 piece of avocado sliced
- 1/4 cup of salsa

Directions:

1. Fry the bacon in a frying pan until it is crisp to taste. Cut it in half, then put aside. Use 2 tsp. of pork fat.

2. Take avocado slices.

3. Beat the eggs in a bowl, and half the cheddar cheese with a whisker. Cook, as you prefer the eggs (scrambled), then remove from the saucepan. Add sea salt and black pepper in the eggs.

4. Position the wraps in the hot skillet, on medium heat, and you can overlap only a little in the center. Separate the scrambled eggs and put them on half of each

cover, not moving halfway through. Add the leftover tomato, bacon, and cheese. Then add one spoonful of water into the pan and immediately cover with a seal.

5. Keep sealed for 1, or 2 minutes, or until the cheese is melted and a little browned off the wraps.

Nutrition:

- Calories: 200
- Proteins: 13g
- Carbs: 2g
- Fat: 15g

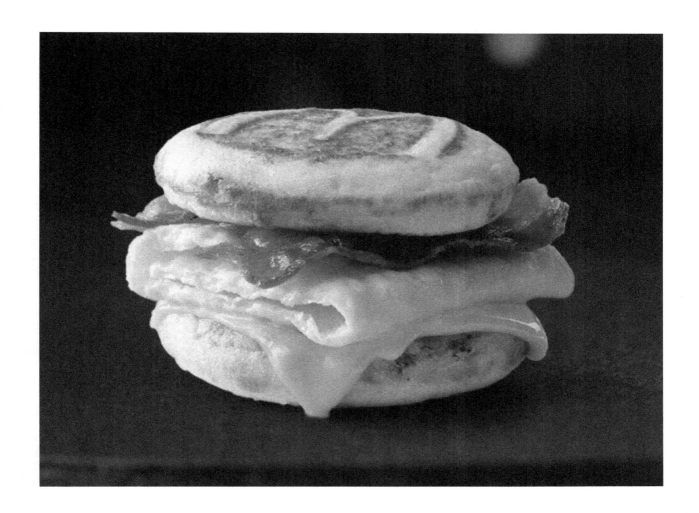

9. MCGriddle Bacon Sandwiches

Preparation Time: 15 Minutes

Cooking Time: 25 Minutes

Servings: 2

Ingredients:

For the Buns:

- 1 cup almond flour (alternative: coconut flour and flaxseed)
- 2 teaspoons baking powder
- ½ teaspoon liquid stevia
- 1 ½ teaspoon erythritol sweetener
- 1 ½ teaspoon vanilla extract, unsweetened
- ½ cup pancake syrup, low-carb, sugar-free
- 3 ounces cream cheese, softened
- 3 eggs

For the Filling:

- 6 slices of bacon, cooked
- ½ teaspoon salt
- ½ teaspoon ground black pepper
- 6 slices of cheese
- 6 eggs

Directions:

1. Take a small saucepan, place it over medium-high heat, add pancake syrup, and bring it to a boil.
2. Continue boiling the syrup for 4 to 8 minutes until reduced by half and thickened, stirring continuously, then spread the syrup on the baking pan lined with parchment paper and let it freeze for 1 hour.
3. Then switch on the oven, set it to 350 °F and let it preheat.

4. Prepare the buns and for this, place all of its remaining ingredients into a blender and then pulse for 2 minutes until smooth.

5. Take a large cookie sheet, line it with a foil, place 12 rings of jars, grease their insides with oil and then evenly pour the blended batter for buns in them, 3 tablespoons per ring.

6. Remove the frozen syrup from the freezer, peel the parchment sheet, then cut syrup into small pieces and evenly spread them out into the batter in the rings.

7. Place the cookie sheet into the oven, bake for 15 minutes until batter for buns has set, and when done, let them cool in the cookie sheet for 5 minutes and then remove buns from the rings to cool completely.

8. Meanwhile, prepare the filling for the buns, and for this, fry the eggs until cooked to the desired level and cook the bacon slices until crisp.

9. Assemble the sandwiches and for this, top each bun with a slice of bacon, a fried egg, a cheese slice, and then cover the top with another bun.

10. Serve straight away.

Nutrition:

- Cal: 374
- Fats: 29 g
- Protein: 19 g
- Net Carb: 2 g
- Fiber: 4 g

10. Kind Bars

Preparation Time: 5 Minutes

Cooking Time: 5 Minutes

Servings: 12

Ingredients:

- 2 cups whole almonds, unsalted
- 2 tablespoons hemp seeds
- ½ cup pumpkin seeds, unsalted
- 2 medium vanilla beans
- 1/3 cup coconut flakes, unsweetened
- ½ teaspoon of sea salt
- ¼ cup erythritol sweetener
- ¼ cup liquid stevia
- 2 teaspoons vanilla extract, unsweetened
- ¼ cup almond butter

Directions:

1. Take a large bowl, place almond, hemp seeds, pumpkin seeds, and coconut flakes in it and then stir until mixed, set aside until required.

2. Take a large saucepan, place it over medium heat, add salt, erythritol, stevia, and butter, and cook for 3 to 5 minutes until smooth, stirring frequently.

3. Remove pan from heat, add vanilla beans and extract, stir until mixed, then spoon the mixture into the almond mixture and stir until combined.

4. Take 8-by-8 inches baking pan, line it with parchment paper, spoon almond mixture in it, spread it evenly by pressing it down, and smooth the top.

5. Cool the almond mixture at room temperature and, when cooled, lift the parchment sheet to transfer the granola to a cutting board and then cut it into bars.

6. Serve straight away.

Nutrition:

- Cal: 216
- Fats: 18 g
- Protein: 8 g
- Net Carb: 3 g
- Fiber: 4 g

Chapter 2: Lunch Keto Recipes

11. Longhorn's Parmesan Crusted Chicken

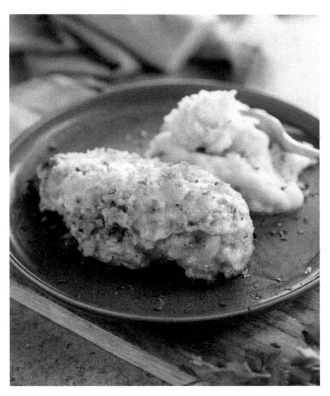

Preparation Time: 10 Minutes

Cooking Time: 30 Minutes

Servings: 4

Ingredients:

- 4 chicken breasts, skinless
- 2 teaspoons salt

- 2 teaspoons ground black pepper
- 2 tablespoons avocado oil

For the Marinade:

- 1 tablespoon minced garlic
- ½ teaspoon ground black pepper
- 1 teaspoon lemon juice
- 3 tablespoon Worcestershire sauce
- 1 teaspoon white vinegar
- ½ cup avocado oil
- ½ cup ranch dressing

For the Parmesan Crust:

- 1 cup panko breadcrumbs
- 6 ounces parmesan cheese, chopped
- 5 tablespoons melted butter, unsalted
- 6 ounces provolone cheese, chopped
- 2 teaspoons garlic powder
- 6 tablespoons ranch salad dressing, low-carb

Directions:

1. Prepare the marinade and for this, take a small bowl, place all of its ingredients in it and then whisk until well combined.

2. Pound each chicken until ¾-inch thick, then season with salt and black pepper and transfer chicken pieces to a large plastic bag.

3. Pour in the prepared marinade, seal the bag, turn it upside to coat chicken with it. For at least 30 minutes, let it stay in the refrigerator.

4. Then take a large skillet pan, place it over medium-high heat, add oil and when hot, place marinated chicken breast in it and then cook for 5 minutes per side until chicken is no longer pink and nicely seared on all sides.

5. Transfer chicken to a plate and repeat with the remaining chicken pieces.

6. Meanwhile, switch on the oven, set it to 450 °F, and let it preheat.

7. When the chicken has cooked, prepare the parmesan crust and for this, take a small heatproof bowl, place both cheeses in it, pour in ranch dressing and milk, stir until mixed, and then microwave for 30 seconds.

8. Then stir the cheese mixture again until smooth and continue microwaving for another 15 seconds.

9. Stir the cheese mixture again, spread evenly on top of each chicken breast, arrange them in a baking sheet and then bake for 5 minutes until cheese has melted.

10. Meanwhile, take a small bowl, place breadcrumbs in it, stir in garlic powder and butter in it.

11. After 5 minutes of baking, spread the breadcrumbs mixture on top of the chicken and then continue baking for 2 minutes until the panko mixture turns light brown.

12. Serve chicken straight away with cauliflower and mashed potatoes.

Nutrition:

- Cal: 557
- Fats: 42 g
- Protein: 31 g
- Net Carb: 10 g
- Fiber: 2 g

12. Panda Express Kung Pao Chicken

Preparation Time: 10 Minutes

Cooking Time: 30 Minutes

Servings: 10

Ingredients:

- 35 ounces chicken thighs, skinless, ½-inch cubed
- 14 ounces zucchini, destemmed, ½-inch diced
- 14 ounces red bell pepper, cored, 1-inch cubed
- 1 green onion, sliced
- 15 pieces of dried Chinese red peppers
- 1 ½ teaspoons minced garlic
- 1 teaspoon minced ginger
- 3 ounces roasted peanuts
- ¼ teaspoon ground black pepper
- ¼ teaspoon xanthan gum
- 3 tablespoons coconut oil
- 1 tablespoon balsamic vinegar
- 1 tablespoon chili garlic sauce
- ¾ tablespoon sesame oil

For the Marinade:

- 3 tablespoons coconut aminos
- 1 tablespoon coconut oil

For the Sauce:

- 3 tablespoons monk fruit sweetener
- 3 tablespoons coconut aminos

Directions:

1. Marinade the chicken and for this, take a large bowl, place the chicken pieces in it, and then add all the ingredients for the marinade in it.

2. Stir until chicken is well coated and then marinate for a minimum of 30 minutes in the refrigerator.

3. Then take a large skillet pan, add 1 tablespoon of coconut oil in it and when it melted, add marinated chicken and cook for 10 minutes or more until it starts to release its water.

4. After 10 minutes, push the chicken to the sides of the pan to create a well in its middle, slowly stir in xanthan gum into the water released by chicken and cook for 2 to 4 minutes until it starts to thicken.

5. Then stir chicken into the thicken liquid and continue cooking for 10 minutes or more until chicken has thoroughly cooked, set aside until required.

6. Return pan over medium-high heat, add 1 tablespoon oil, and when it melts, add bell pepper and zucchini cubes and then cook for 5 to 8 minutes until lightly browned.

7. Transfer vegetables to a separate plate, then add remaining coconut oil into the pan, add Chinese red peppers, ginger, garlic, vinegar, and chili garlic sauce.

8. Stir until mixed, cook for 3 minutes, add ingredients for the sauce along with peanuts, green onion, black pepper, and sesame oil and continue cooking for 3 minutes, stirring frequently.

9. Return chicken and vegetables into the pan, toss until well mixed and then continue cooking for 3 to 5 minutes until hot.

10. Serve straight away.

Nutrition:

- Cal: 295
- Fats: 16.4 g
- Protein: 31.7 g
- Net Carb: 3.2 g
- Fiber: 2 g

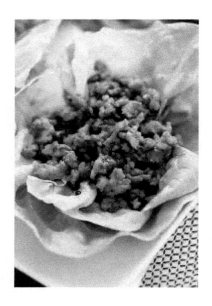

13. Chang's Lettuce Wraps

Preparation Time: 10 Minutes

Cooking Time: 15 Minutes

Servings: 8

Ingredients:

For the Sauce:

- 1 tablespoon minced garlic
- ½ teaspoon grated ginger
- 1 tablespoon Swerve sweetener

- 3 tablespoons soy sauce
- 1 tablespoon apple cider vinegar
- 1 tablespoon almond butter

For the Wraps:

- 1 pound ground chicken
- 3 ounces chopped shiitake mushrooms
- 3 green onions, sliced
- 2 teaspoons onion powder
- ½ cup diced jicama
- ¼ teaspoon salt
- ¼ teaspoon ground black pepper
- 1 tablespoon avocado oil
- 1 large head of butter lettuce

Directions:

1. Prepare the sauce and for this, take a medium bowl, place all of its ingredients in it and then whisk until combined, set aside until required.

2. Take a large skillet pan, place it over medium heat, add oil and when hot, add ground chicken, crumble it and then cook for 5 to 8 minutes until no longer pink.

3. Season chicken with salt, onion powder, and black pepper, add mushrooms, green onion, and jicama and then cook for 5 minutes until mushrooms have turned softened.

4. Pour in the prepared sauce, stir until combined, cook for 2 minutes until hot, and then remove the pan from heat.

5. Divide lettuce leaves into 16 portions, top each with ¼ cup of the chicken and then serve straight away.

Nutrition:

- Cal: 149
- Fats: 9 g
- Protein: 12 g
- Net Carb: 2.5 g
- Fiber: 2 g

14. Asian Chicken Taco Lettuce Wraps

Preparation Time: 15 Minutes

Cooking Time: 20 Minutes

Servings: 4

Ingredients:

For the Chicken:

- 1 tablespoon minced garlic
- 1 pound chicken thighs, skinless, boneless
- 2 tablespoons taco seasoning
- 1 tablespoon avocado oil

For the Wrap:

- 1 large avocado, peeled, pitted, diced
- ¼ cup diced white onion
- 8 leaves of romaine lettuce
- 1 medium tomato, diced

For the Cilantro Sauce:

- 1 jalapeno pepper
- ½ teaspoon minced garlic
- ½ cup cilantro leaves

- ½ of lime, juiced
- ¼ teaspoon salt
- ½ cup sour cream
- 2 tablespoons avocado oil

Directions:

1. Prepare the chicken and for this, place chicken in a large plastic bag, add remaining ingredients into it, seal the bag and shake well until chicken is well coated.
2. Place the bag into the refrigerator and then let it marinate for a minimum of 30 minutes.
3. Then take a griddle pan, place it over medium-high heat, grease it with oil and when hot, place marinated chicken on it and cook for 10 minutes per side until cooked and nicely browned.
4. While chicken marinates, prepare the cilantro sauce and for this, place all of its ingredients in a food processor and then pulse for 1 minute until blended; set aside until required.
5. Assemble the wraps and for this, distribute chicken among lettuce leaves, then top with onion, avocado and tomatoes, and drizzle with prepared cilantro sauce.
6. Serve straight away.

Nutrition:

- Cal: 161
- Fats: 9.1 g
- Protein: 14.5 g
- Net Carb: 4.9 g
- Fiber: 1.2 g

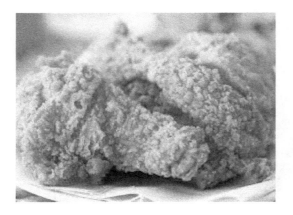

15. KFC Fried Chicken

Preparation Time: 15 Minutes

Cooking Time: 18 Minutes

Servings: 6

Ingredients:

For the Seasoning:

- 1 teaspoon celery salt
- 1 teaspoon of sea salt
- 1 teaspoon ginger powder
- 1 tablespoon ground white pepper
- 2 teaspoons garlic salt
- 1 teaspoon ground black pepper

- 4 teaspoons paprika
- ¼ teaspoon dried oregano
- ½ teaspoon dried thyme
- 1 teaspoon mustard powder

For the Marinade:

- ½ of the seasoning
- 4 tablespoons white vinegar
- 3 tablespoons heavy cream
- 2 cups almond milk, unsweetened
- 2 eggs

For the Chicken:

- 8 ½ cups avocado oil
- 2 pounds of chicken drumsticks
- 2 ½ cups whey protein powder

Directions:

1. Prepare the seasoning and for this, take a small bowl, place all of its ingredients in it and then stir until mixed, set aside until required.
2. Prepare the marinade and for this, take a large bowl, pour in milk, add vinegar and cream, whisk until blended and then let it sit for 10 minutes.
3. Then whisk in eggs until combined, and whisk in ½ of seasoning until smooth.
4. Place chicken pieces into a large plastic bag, pour in the marinade, seal the bag, turn it upside down to coat chicken and then let it marinate in the refrigerator for a minimum of 4 hours.

5. Cook the chicken, and for this, take a large pan, place it over medium heat, pour in the oil, and heat it for 12 minutes or more until the temperature reaches 325 °F.

6. Spread remaining seasoning mixture on a plate, take a chicken piece, coat it with the seasoning mix and then add into the pan.

7. Add more seasoned chicken pieces into the pan until filled and cook for 16 to 18 minutes until the internal temperature of chicken reaches 165 °F and turns nicely browned, turning chicken frequently.

8. When done, transfer fried chicken to a plate lined with paper towels, and then repeat with the remaining chicken pieces.

9. Serve straight away.

Nutrition:

- Cal 590.2
- Fats 39.6 g
- Protein 57.6 g
- Net Carb 1.1 g
- Fiber 1 g

16. Tso's Shrimp and Broccoli

Preparation Time: 5 Minutes

Cooking Time: 20 Minutes

Servings: 4

Ingredients:

- 1 large head of broccoli, cut into florets
- 1-pound medium shrimp, tails removed, peeled, deveined
- ½ tablespoon minced garlic
- 1 teaspoon of sea salt
- ½ teaspoon ground black pepper
- 1 tablespoon crushed red pepper
- 2 tablespoons monk fruit sweetener
- 2 tablespoons white vinegar
- 3 tablespoons liquid aminos
- 2 tablespoons avocado oil
- 1/3 cup ketchup, sugar-free
- 1 teaspoon toasted sesame seeds

Directions:

1. Take a large bowl, place broccoli florets in it, cover with a plastic wrap, microwave for 10 minutes or more until florets have steamed, and then drain them well.

2. Meanwhile, take a medium bowl, place the shrimps in it and then season with salt and black pepper.

3. Prepare the sauce and for this, take a small saucepan, place it over medium heat, add garlic, sweetener, ketchup, soy sauce, and vinegar and then stir until mixed.

4. Bring the mixture to a boil and then remove the pan from heat.

5. Take a large skillet pan, place it over medium-high heat, add oil and when hot, add seasoned shrimps, and then cook for 5 to 8 minutes until turned pink.

6. Drizzle with sauce, toss well until coated, and stir-fry for 3 to 5 minutes until shrimps have caramelized slightly.

7. When done, remove the pan from heat and garnish shrimps with sesame seeds.

8. Distribute the broccoli florets among 4 plates, top with shrimps, and then serve.

Nutrition:

- Cal: 443
- Fats: 18 g
- Protein: 54 g
- Net Carb: 2 g
- Fiber: 2 g

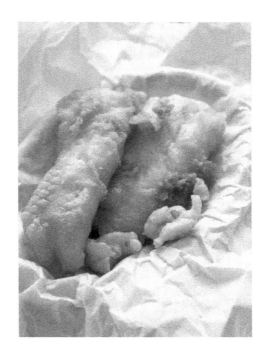

17. Long John Silver's Batter-Dipped Fish

Preparation Time: 5 Minutes

Cooking Time: 10 Minutes

Servings: 6

Ingredients:

- 4 cups vegetable oil (for frying)
- 2 pounds cod (cut into three-inch pieces)
- 16 ounces club soda

- ¼ cup ground flaxseed
- 2 cups almond flour
- ½ teaspoon paprika
- ½ teaspoon onion salt
- ½ teaspoon baking soda
- ½ teaspoon baking powder
- 1 teaspoon Himalayan sea salt
- ¼ teaspoon black pepper

Directions:

1. First, take a deep-frying pan and fill it with the 4 cups of oil. Turn the heat to medium to preheat the oil.

2. As the oil heats, combine the almond flour and ground flaxseed with the paprika, onion salt, baking soda, baking powder, sea salt, and black pepper into a medium-sized mixing bowl. Whisk everything together so it is well incorporated, then add the club soda. Whisk again until the batter has a foamy consistency.

3. Take the cod pieces and dip them into the batter. Ensure that each piece is coated completely, then carefully place them into the preheated oil. Do not overcrowd the pan or the fish will not cook evenly. If needed, fry in 2 batches. Allow the fish to fry for 5 minutes. The fish should have a nice golden color and will begin to float on the oil when done.

4. Remove the fish from the oil using a slotted spoon and transfer them to a plate lined with paper towels to catch the excess oil.

5. Serve with your favorite side!

Nutrition:

- Calories: 559

- Carbs: 2g
- Fat: 43g
- Protein: 37g

18. Olive Garden's Steak Gorgonzola Alfredo

Preparation Time: 20 Minutes

Cooking Time: 25 Minutes

Servings: 4

Ingredients:

- 1 pound of steak medallions
- 1 tablespoon balsamic vinegar
- ½ teaspoon Himalayan sea salt
- ½ teaspoon black pepper
- 5 zucchinis
- 4 ounces gorgonzola crumbles
- ¼ cup sun-dried tomatoes

For the Sauce

- 2 cups heavy cream
- 1 stick of unsalted butter
- 1 cup parmesan cheese
- 2 cups spinach
- ¼ teaspoon nutmeg
- ¼ teaspoon Himalayan sea salt

- ¼ teaspoon black pepper

Directions:

1. Begin by marinating your steaks. First, sprinkle them with the Himalayan sea salt and black pepper, then place them in a sealable bag. Add the balsamic vinegar to the bag and seal. Place the steaks in the refrigerator for at least 30 minutes before cooking

2. As the steaks marinate, place a large pot of water on the stovetop and turn the heat to medium high. Then take a spiralizer and create the "fettuccine noodles" using the zucchini. You can also use a vegetable peeler to peel thicker zoodles if you do not have a spiralizer. When done, add them to the boiling pot of water for 3 minutes. Then, drain the water and transfer the zucchini noodles to a plate lined with a paper towel, so the excess water can drain off.

3. Next, take a large skillet and place it on the stove. Turn the heat to medium and allow it to heat up. Remove the steak medallions and place them into the hot skillet. Allow them to cook on each side for about five minutes. The thickness of the steak will determine how long you need to cook the steaks. Steaks that are a little over 2 inches should reach a medium cook in 5 minutes per side. If you prefer the steak rarer, cook for a shorter amount of time. For those who like a more well-done steak, cook for 2 minutes longer. Your steaks should have a nice brown color when they are done.

4. Once the steaks have reached your desired cook time, remove them from the skillet and place them on a plate, then cover them with aluminum foil to rest. Keep in mind the steaks will still continue to cook even though you have removed them from the skillet.

5. As the steaks rest, you want to make the sauce. Place a medium-sized saucepan on the stove and turn the heat to medium. Add in the butter and heavy cream. Once the butter has begun to melt, add in the spinach. Allow the spinach to cook down; this should only take about 5 minutes. Once the spinach has wilted, add in the parmesan cheese, sea salt, and black pepper. Stir, reduce heat to medium low and allow the sauce to thicken slightly for about 5 minutes.

6. Once the sauce is done, turn off the heat. Transfer your zucchini noodles to a large bowl and pour the sauce over top (leave a little sauce in the saucepan to top your steaks with). Toss the zucchini noodles with the sauce so that everything gets

nicely coated. Add in the gorgonzola cheese, but reserve some to top your steaks with during plating. Toss everything one more time.

7. Now it is time to assemble the plate! Place a small portion of the zucchini noodles on your dinner plate, place a steak medallion on top of the noodles, and top with the dried tomatoes, gorgonzola crumbles, and a little drizzle of your leftover sauce.

Nutrition:

- Calories: 413
- Carbs: 6g
- Fat: 28g
- Protei: 30g

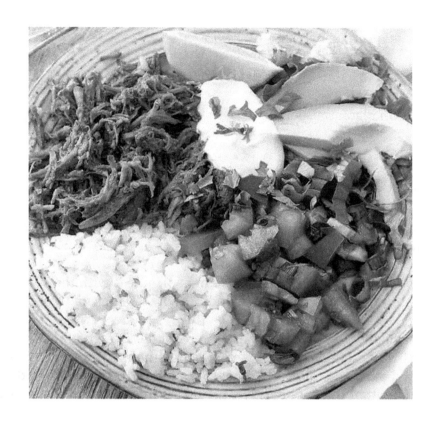

19. Chipotle's Chipotle Pork Carnitas

Preparation Time: 5 Minutes

Cooking Time: 4 Hours 10 Minutes

Servings: 8

Ingredients:

- 1 cup water
- 2 tablespoons avocado oil

- 4 pounds pork roast
- 1 teaspoon thyme
- 2 teaspoon juniper berries
- 1 teaspoon Himalayan sea salt
- ½ teaspoon black pepper

Directions:

1. Begin by preheating your oven to 300 °Fahrenheit.
2. Next, take a Dutch oven pot, place it on the stove, and turn the heat to medium. Add the avocado oil to the pot.
3. As the pot heats, take the pork roast and sprinkle it with the sea salt. Then place the roast into the Dutch oven pot and brown the sides for a minute on each side.
4. Turn the heat off on the stove once the roast has browned. Add the water, thyme, juniper berries, and black pepper to the pot, then cover. Place the pot into the preheated oven and allow the roast to cook for 3 ½ hours. Turn the roast every half hour so that the flavors really penetrate into all areas of the meat.
5. Remove the roast from the oven after 3 ½ hours (keep the oven turned on), allow it to rest for 10 minutes, then use two forks to pull the meat apart. Once all the meat has been pulled, place the pot back into the oven for 30 minutes.
6. Remove the pot and enjoy!

Nutrition:

- Calories: 317
- Carbs: .5g
- Fat: 14.5g
- Protein: 43g

20. Red Lobster's Shrimp Scampi with Cheddar Bay Biscuits

Preparation Time: 10 Minutes

Cooking Time: 25 Minutes

Servings: 4

Ingredients:

For the Scampi:

- 1 ¼ pounds shrimp (peeled, tail removed, deveined)
- 2 garlic cloves (minced)
- 2 scallions (sliced)
- 4 tablespoons butter (unsalted)
- 1/3 cup parmesan cheese (shredded)
- ¼ cup lemon juice
- ¼ cup chardonnay
- ¼ cup parsley (chopped)
- ¼ teaspoon red pepper flakes

For the Biscuits:

- 1 ½ cups almond flour
- 2 eggs
- 1 ½ teaspoons garlic powder (separated into 1 and then ½ teaspoon)

- 1 tablespoon baking powder
- ½ cup cheddar cheese (shredded)
- ½ cup sour cream
- 6 tablespoons butter (unsalted, melted, separated into 4 and then 2 tablespoons)
- 1 tablespoon parsley (minced)
- ½ teaspoon Himalayan sea salt

Directions:

1. Place a large skillet on the stove and turn the heat to medium with the butter in it. Allow the skillet to heat up for a few minutes until the butter has melted, then add the garlic. Cook the garlic for 1 minute so that it becomes a light golden color.

2. Take the shrimps and add them to the skillet. Let them cook for 3 minutes. Sprinkle the red pepper flake over the shrimp, flip, and cook for another 3 minutes.

3. Once the shrimps have turned a pink color, pour in the lemon juice and chardonnay. Allow everything to simmer for 2 minutes, then turn off the heat.

4. Add the scallion and parsley to the skillet. Stir everything together and top with the parmesan cheese.

5. Serve over top of your favorite vegetable noodles like zucchini or spaghetti squash.

To make the Biscuits:

1. Preheat your oven to 450 °F., then grease a muffin pan with oil and set to the side.

2. In a large mixing bowl, add the almond flour, 1 teaspoon of garlic, baking powder, and salt. Use a fork to mix everything together, set to the side.

3. In a small bowl, crack your eggs, then pour in 4 tablespoons of the melted butter and the sour cream. Beat the eggs and sour cream until well incorporated, then

add to the flour mixture. Stir the ingredients together until you have a smooth batter, then fold in the cheddar cheese.

4. Take the muffin pan and fill each segment with the batter. Place the pan into the oven and bake for 10 minutes. The biscuits should be a light golden color when they are done. Ensure the inside of the biscuits are done by inserting a wooden toothpick into one. If it comes out clean, they are done. If there is batter coated on the toothpick, put them back into the oven for a few more minutes.

5. As the biscuits bake, take a small bowl and add the remaining 2 tablespoons of butter and ½ teaspoon of garlic powder. Stir together until the garlic powder has dissolved, then add the parsley. Once the biscuits have been removed from the oven, brush each one with the butter and parsley mixture, then serve warm.

Nutrition:

- Calories: 591
- Carbs: 6g
- Fat: 39g
- Protein: 45g

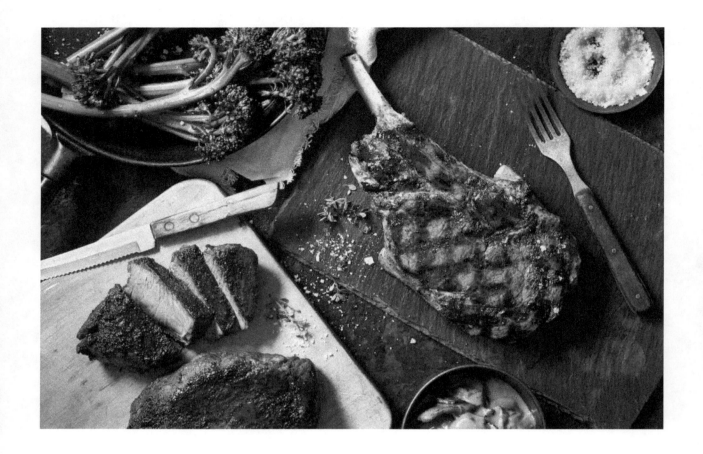

21. Outback Steakhouse Charcoal Ribeye

Preparation Time: 5 Minutes

Cooking Time: 15 Minutes

Servings: 8

Ingredients:

- 4 ribeye steaks (cut to 1 ½-inch thick slices, fat trimmed)

- 1 teaspoon turmeric powder
- 2 teaspoons paprika
- 1 teaspoon chili powder
- ½ teaspoon thyme (dried)
- ½ teaspoon garlic powder
- ½ teaspoon onion powder
- ½ teaspoon ground mustard
- ½ teaspoon cumin (ground)
- ½ teaspoon ancho chili pepper (ground)
- ½ teaspoon Himalayan sea salt
- ½ teaspoon black pepper

Directions:

1. Begin by placing a grill pan on the stove or turn the outdoor grill on to medium-high heat. Brush the grill pan or outdoor grill with oil.

2. Next, take a small bowl and combine the turmeric powder, paprika, chili powder, thyme, garlic powder, onion powder, ground mustard, cumin, ancho chili pepper, sea salt, and black pepper. Use a fork to thoroughly mix all the ingredients together.

3. Take each of your steaks and season them generously with the spice mixture on both sides. Then place the steaks onto the grill. Cook for 5 minutes on each side for a medium-cooked steak. Remove the steaks from the grill when they are at your desired doneness and cover them with foil to rest for 5 minutes.

4. When the steaks have rested, slice the steaks and serve on top of your favorite salad or along with your favorite roasted vegetables.

Nutrition:

- Calories: 139
- Carbs: 2g
- Fat: 4g
- Protein: 27g

22. Chicken Pan with Veggies and Pesto

Preparation Time: 10 Minutes

Cooking Time: 20 Minutes

Servings: 4

Ingredients:

- 2 Tbsp. olive oil
- 1 lb. chicken thighs, boneless, skinless, sliced into strips
- ¾ cup oil-packed sun-dried tomatoes, chopped
- 1 pound asparagus ends
- ¼ cup basil pesto
- 1 cup cherry tomatoes, red and yellow, halved
- Salt, to taste

Directions:

1. Heat olive oil in a frying pan over medium-high heat.
2. Put salt on the chicken slices and then put it into a skillet, add the sun-dried tomatoes and fry for 5–10 minutes. Remove the chicken slices and season with salt. Add asparagus to the skillet. Cook for additional 5–10 minutes.
3. Then, place the chicken back in the skillet, pour in the pesto, and whisk. Fry for 1–2 minutes. Remove from the heat. Add the halved cherry tomatoes and pesto. Stir well and serve.

Nutrition:

- Carbohydrates: 12 g

- Fat: 32 g
- Protein: 2 g
- Calories: 423

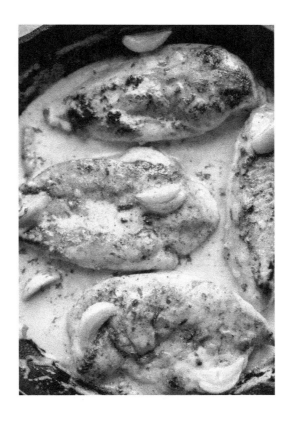

23. Creamy Garlic Chicken

Preparation Time: 5 Minutes

Cooking Time: 15 Minutes

Servings: 4

Ingredients:

- 4 chicken breasts, finely sliced
- 1 tsp garlic powder

- 1 tsp paprika
- 2 Tbsp. butter
- 1 tsp salt
- 1 cup heavy cream
- ½ cup sun-dried tomatoes
- 2 garlic cloves, minced
- 1 cup spinach, chopped

Directions:

1. Blend the paprika, garlic powder, and salt and sprinkle over both sides of the chicken.

2. Melt the butter in a frying pan (choose medium heat). Add the chicken breast and fry for 5 minutes each side. Set aside.

3. Add the heavy cream, sun-dried tomatoes, and garlic to the pan and whisk well to combine. Cook for 2 minutes. Add spinach and sauté for an additional 3 minutes. Return the chicken to the pan and cover with the sauce.

Nutrition:

- Carbohydrates: 12 g
- Fat: 26 g
- Protein: 4 g
- Calories: 280

24. Chinese Pork Bowl

Preparation Time: 5 Minutes

Cooking Time: 15 Minutes

Servings: 4

Ingredients:

- Salt and ground black pepper, to taste
- 1¼ pounds pork belly, cut into bite-size pieces
- 2 Tbsp. tamari soy sauce
- 1 Tbsp. Rice vinegar
- 2 garlic cloves, smashed
- 3 oz. butter
- 1 pound Brussels sprouts, rinsed, trimmed, halved or quartered
- ½ leek, chopped

Directions:

1. Fry the pork over medium-high heat until it is starting to turn golden brown.
2. Combine the garlic cloves, butter, and Brussel sprouts. Add to the pan, whisk well and cook until the sprouts turn golden brown.
3. Stir the soy sauce and rice vinegar together and pour the sauce into the pan.
4. Sprinkle with salt and pepper.
5. Top with chopped leek.

Nutrition:

- Carbohydrates: 7 g
- Fat: 97 g
- Protein: 19 g
- Calories: 993

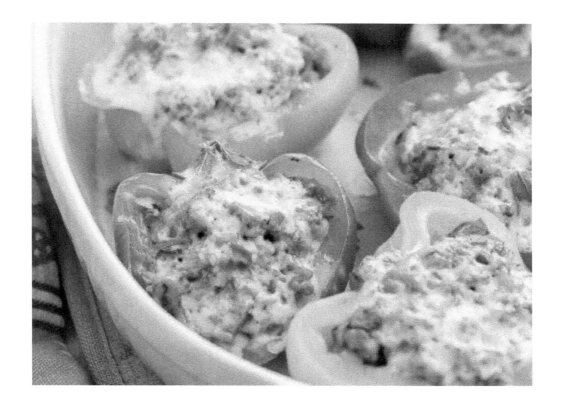

25. Turkey-Pepper Mix

Preparation Time: 5 Minutes

Cooking Time: 20 Minutes

Servings: 1

Ingredients:

- 1 pound turkey tenderloin, cut into thin steaks
- 1 tsp salt, divided

- 2 Tbsp. extra-virgin olive oil, divided
- ½ sweet onion, sliced
- 1 red bell pepper, cut into strips
- 1 yellow bell pepper, cut into strips
- ½ tsp Italian seasoning
- ¼ tsp ground black pepper
- 2 tsp red wine vinegar
- 1 14-ounces crushed tomatoes, roasted Fresh parsley Basil

Directions:

1. Sprinkle ½ tsp of salt on your turkey. Pour 1 Tbsp. of oil into the pan and heat it. Add the turkey steaks and cook for 1–3 minutes per side. Set aside.

2. Put the onion, bell peppers, and the remaining salt to the pan and cook for 7 minutes, stirring all the time. Sprinkle with Italian seasoning and add black pepper. Cook for 30 seconds. Add the tomatoes and vinegar and fry the mix for about 20 seconds.

3. Now, return the turkey to the pan and pour the sauce over it. Simmer for 2–3 minutes.

4. Top with chopped parsley and basil.

Nutrition:

- Carbohydrates: 11 g
- Fat: 8 g
- Protein: 30 g
- Calories: 230

26. Simple Tuna Salad

Preparation Time: 5 Minutes

Cooking Time: 0 Minutes

Servings: 4

Ingredients:

- 10 oz. canned tuna, drained
- 1 avocado, chopped
- 1 rib celery, chopped
- 2 fresh garlic cloves, minced
- 3 Tbsp. Mayonnaise
- 1 red onion, chopped
- 1 Tbsp. lemon juice
- 8 sprigs parsley
- ¼ cucumber, chopped Salt and pepper, to taste

Directions:

1. Divide the parsley into 2 halves.
2. And then, mix all the ingredients, except half of the parsley, in a separate bowl. Stir well.
3. Add salt and pepper to taste.
4. Top with the remaining parsley.

Nutrition:

- Carbohydrates: 1.7 g
- Fat: 16.3 g
- Protein: 13.9 g
- Calories: 225

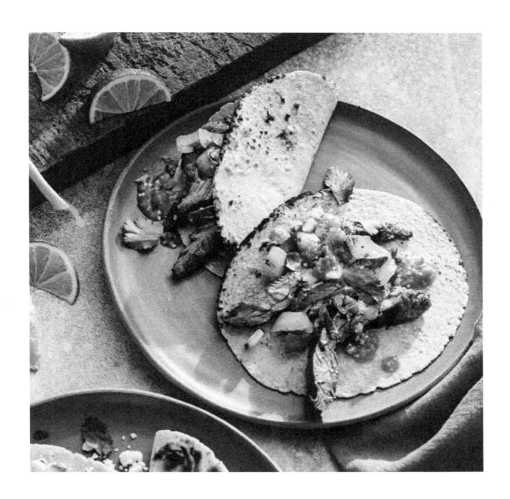

27. Chipotle Steak with Tortilla

Preparation Time: 5 Minutes

Cooking Time: 15 Minutes

Servings: 4

Ingredients:

- 16 oz. skirt steak
- 4 oz. pepper jack cheese
- 1 cup sour cream
- 1 handful fresh cilantro
- 1 tbsp. extra virgin olive oil
- 1 splash chipotle tabasco sauce
- Salt and pepper to taste

Homemade Guacamole

- 2 avocados(s)
- 2 tsp lime juice
- 2 tbsps. Fresh cilantro
- Salt and pepper to taste

Directions:

1. Season the skirt steak to taste with salt and pepper.
2. Then, on high heat, heat a cast iron skillet.
3. Then, add olive oil when the skillet is hot and cook the skirt steak for around 4 minutes on each side.
4. Now, place it on a plate to rest while you prepare the guacamole.
5. Slice the steak against the grain and make it into bite-sized strips. Divide the same into 4 equal portions.
6. Add the cheese to the top portion. Follow that with ¼ cup of guacamole and ¼ cup of sour cream.

7. Splash each portion with some chipotle tabasco sauce (not necessary) and fresh cilantro.

8. Prepare the guacamole and serve with low carb tortillas. For homemade guacamole, remove the pit from the avocado and then mash the content. Add the rest of the ingredients and serve.

Nutrition:

- Calories: 810
- Fat: 61g
- Carbohydrates: 15g
- Fiber: 11.5g
- Net carbs: 3.5g
- Protein: 34g

28. Bacon-Wrapped Chicken Breast

Preparation Time: 10 Minutes

Cooking Time: 45 Minutes

Servings: 4

Ingredients:

- 4 boneless, skinless chicken breasts
- 8 oz. sharp cheddar cheese
- 8 slices bacon
- 4 oz. sliced jalapeno peppers
- 1 tsp garlic powder
- Salt and pepper to taste

Directions:

1. Preheat the oven at around 350ºF.
2. Ensure to season both sides of chicken breast well with salt, garlic powder, and pepper.
3. Place the chicken breast on a non-stick baking sheet (foil-covered).
4. Cover the chicken with cheese and add jalapeno slices.
5. Cut the bacon slices in half and then place the 4 halves over each piece of chicken.
6. Bake for around 30 to 45 minutes at most.
7. If the chicken is set, but the bacon still feels undercooked, you may want to put it under the broiler for a few minutes.

8. Once done, serve hot with a side of low carb garlic parmesan roasted asparagus.

Nutrition:

- Calories: 640
- Fat: 48g
- Carbohydrates: 6g
- Fiber: 3g
- Net carbs: 3g
- Protein: 47g

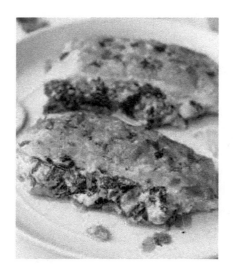

29. Spinach Stuffed Salmon

Preparation Time: 10 Minutes

Cooking Time: 15 Minutes

Servings: 4

Ingredients:

- 24 oz. salmon filets
- 2 tbsps. Extra virgin olive oil
- 2 tbsps. Grass-fed butter
- 1/4 tsp garlic powder
- Salt and pepper to taste

Low Carb Spinach Dip

- 2 tbsps. Grass-fed butter
- 12 oz. baby spinach
- 8 oz. of cream cheese
- ½ cup Asiago cheese (shredded)
- 1 minced garlic clove
- Salt and pepper

Directions:

1. Cut the salmon into 4 6-ounce pieces. Make a slit in each part of the salmon to create pockets using a paring knife.
2. Now, season the entire salmon with salt, garlic powder, and pepper.
3. For the stuffing, we need to make a low carb spinach dip. For that, add spinach, garlic, salt, butter, and pepper to a sauté pan—Cook for around 5 minutes.
4. Add cream cheese while the spinach is cooling along with asiago cheese in a mixing bowl. Mix nicely until no lumps remain.
5. Add the spinach to the mixture.
6. Use the pockets we made earlier and stuff low carb spinach dip mixture.
7. Now, add olive oil to a large sauté pan and then add the salmon, skin-down, and cook for 6-8 mins. Until skin is crispy. Flip the salmon and cook for another 6 to 8 minutes.
8. Once done, remove salmon from the pan, add butter and serve.

Nutrition:

- Calories: 336

- Fat: 23g

- Carbohydrates: 0g

- Fiber: 0g

- Net carbs: 0g

- Protein: 33g

30. Creamy Zoodles

Preparation Time: 2 Minutes

Cooking Time: 3 Minutes

Servings: 1

Ingredients:

- 3 minced garlic cloves
- 2 tablespoons of butter
- 2 medium zucchinis
- 1/4 teaspoon salt to taste
- 1/4 teaspoon pepper
- 1/4 cup of parmesan cheese

Directions:

1. Wash the zucchini, then cut it to strands using a spiralizer or vegetable peeler; and then set aside. If done right, the zucchini should come out like spaghetti strands. I mean, that's the point, right?

2. Put a large pan on medium heat. Put the butter in to melt and then add minced garlic. Stir-fry the garlic until it starts to appear translucent. If you know you have an affinity for burning things, please be attentive so the garlic doesn't get burnt.

3. Add the zucchini strands and stir fry for 3 minutes. Make sure to taste the noodle strands to check how tender they are as zucchini cooks really fast. Try not to "taste" till it finishes.

4. Bring down the pan, add salt, pepper and parmesan cheese, stir until well combined and serve.

Nutrition:

- Calories: 100
- Total Fat: 4g
- Carbs: 4g
- Protein: 4g

Chapter 3: Dinner Keto Recipes

31. Creamy Chicken and Mushroom Casserole

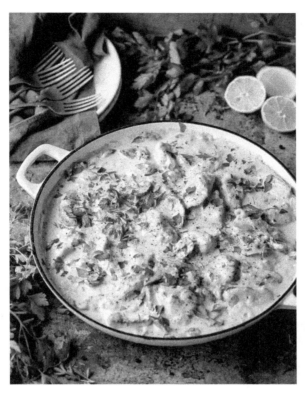

Preparation Time: 5 Minutes

Cooking Time: 10 Minutes

Servings: 8

Ingredients:

- 2 pounds chicken tenderloin
- 4 tablespoons butter

- 4 garlic cloves, crushed
- ¼ cup fresh thyme leaves
- 1-pound mushrooms, cut into thick slices
- 4 tablespoons olive oil
- ½ cup chopped fresh parsley
- Salt to taste
- Pepper to taste
- 1 cup heavy cream
- 1 cup chicken stock
- ½ cup sour cream

Directions:

1. Add 2 tablespoons oil and 2 tablespoons butter into a heavy skillet.
2. Place the skillet over medium flame. Let the butter melt.
3. Place chicken in the skillet and sprinkle salt and pepper. Fry until brown all over. Cook in batches if required.
4. Remove chicken and place it on a plate.
5. Add retained oil and butter into the skillet. Let the butter melt. Add mushrooms and cook until brown.
6. Add garlic, stock, and fresh herbs and mix well. Remove any browned bits that may be stuck on the bottom of the pan by scraping with a spatula.
7. Stir in the sour cream and cream and simmer until it begins to bubble slightly.
8. Add chicken and stir until well coated. Let it simmer for about 5 to 6 minutes.

9. Turn off the heat. Cover and let it sit for 10 minutes.

10. Serve. Any remaining casserole can be placed in an airtight container in the refrigerator for 5 days.

Nutrition:

- Calories: 400
- Fat: 29 g
- Total Carbohydrate: 5 g
- Digestible carbohydrate: 4 g
- Edible fibers: 1 g
- Protein: 27 g

32. Skillet Chicken Florentine

Preparation Time: 5 Minutes

Cooking Time: 30 Minutes

Servings: 2

Ingredients:

- 2 chicken thighs, bone-in, skin on
- 6 tablespoons chicken stock
- ¼ teaspoon Himalayan pink salt
- ¼ teaspoon Italian seasoning or to taste
- ¼ teaspoon garlic powder
- Pepper to taste
- ¼ teaspoon onion powder
- 1 tablespoon avocado oil
- ½ cup heavy whipping cream
- 4 ounces cremini mushrooms, sliced
- 1 ½ cups chopped spinach
- 6 tablespoons shredded parmesan cheese

Directions:

1. Heat a cast iron skillet over medium flame. Add the oil, and once it's heated, add chicken and cook until the skin is golden brown and the chicken is nearly cooked through.

2. Take out the chicken and set aside in a bowl.

3. Pour stock and whipping cream into the skillet. Add spices and stir.

4. When the mixture begins to simmer, lower the heat and add mushrooms.

5. Cook until mushrooms are soft. Stir in parmesan and spinach. Cook until spinach wilts.

6. Add the chicken and simmer until the chicken is well cooked. Stir occasionally.

7. Serve hot.

Nutrition:

- Calories: 668
- Fat: 2 g
- Total Carbohydrate: 12 g
- Digestible carbohydrate: 8 g
- Edible fibers: 4 g
- Protein: 45 g

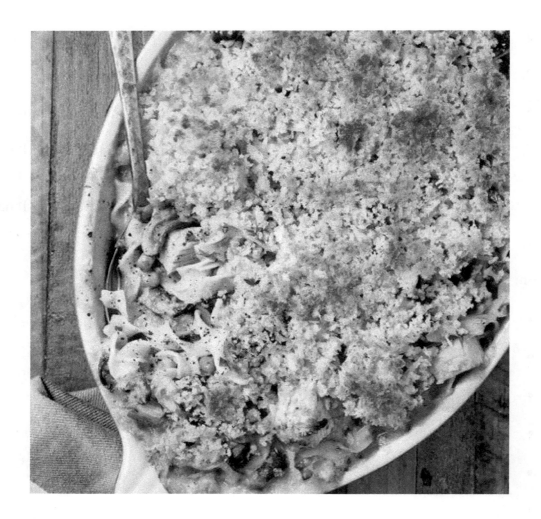

33. Turkey Casserole

Preparation Time: 5 Minutes

Cooking Time: 30 Minutes

Servings: 4

Ingredients:

- 11.11 ounces turkey breast, cooked, shredded (or use leftovers)
- ¾ cup green beans
- ¼ small onion, sliced
- 4 brown mushrooms, sliced
- ½ small carrot, chopped
- 3 garlic cloves, peeled, sliced
- 2 tablespoons butter
- 1 tablespoon chopped parsley
- ½ cup broccoli florets
- ½ cup shredded cheddar cheese
- 1 tablespoon crushed pork rinds

For keto white sauce:

- 1 tablespoon butter
- ¾ cup heavy cream
- ½ teaspoon salt
- 3.5 ounces cream cheese, cut into small cubes
- ¼ cup shredded parmesan cheese
- Pepper to taste
- 1/8 teaspoon nutmeg

Directions:

1. Place a pot over medium flame. Add butter. When butter melts, add garlic, onions, and carrots and sauté for a couple of minutes.

2. Cover and cook for another 2 minutes.

3. Uncover and stir in the broccoli and mushrooms. Stir-fry for a minute.

4. Cover again and cook for 2 more minutes.

5. Stir in the turkey. Remove from heat.

6. To make sauce: Place a small pot over medium flame. Add butter and cream cheese and whisk until cream cheese melts. The butter and cream cheese will not combine.

7. Stir in the heavy cream. Remove from heat. Spoon sauce over the turkey mixture and stir.

8. Spread the turkey mixture into a casserole dish.

9. Top with grated cheese. Scatter parsley and pork rinds on top.

10. Bake in a preheated oven at 300ºF for about 20 to 30 minutes until golden brown.

Nutrition:

- Calories: 510
- Fat: 40.98 g
- Total Carbohydrate: 8.64 g
- Digestible carbohydrate: 6.84 g
- Edible fibers: 1.8 g
- Protein: 28.72 g

34. Turkey with Cream-Cheese Sauce

Preparation Time: 5 Minutes

Cooking Time: 30 Minutes

Servings: 8

Ingredients:

- 3 pounds turkey breast
- 4 tablespoons butter
- 4 cups heavy whipping cream
- Salt to taste
- Pepper to taste
- 2 tablespoons tamari
- 14 ounces cream cheese
- 2/3 cup small capers

Directions:

1. Place a large ovenproof skillet over medium flame. Add half the butter and melt.
2. Sprinkle salt and pepper liberally over the turkey and place in the skillet.
3. Cook until brown all over.
4. Transfer the skillet into a preheated oven.
5. Roast at 350°F for about 30 minutes or the internal temperature of the meat is 165°F.

6. Remove turkey from the oven and place it on the cutting board. Cover turkey with foil loosely and let it rest for a while. When cool enough to handle, cut into slices.

7. Transfer the cooked liquid from the skillet into a saucepan. Place the saucepan over medium flame. Stir in the heavy cream and cream cheese.

8. Reduce the heat to low heat and cook until thick. Add tamari, salt, and pepper and stir. Turn off the heat.

9. Place a pan over high flame. Add butter. When butter melts, add capers and cook until crisp.

10. To assemble: Place turkey slices on a large serving platter. Pour sauce over turkey. Garnish with fried capers and serve.

Nutrition:

- Calories: 815
- Fat: 67 g
- Total Carbohydrate: 7 g
- Digestible carbohydrate: 7 g
- Edible fibers: 0 g
- Protein: 47 g

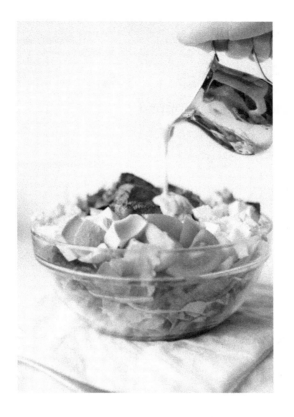

35. Steak Cobb Salad with Cilantro Lime Vinaigrette

Preparation Time: 5 Minutes

Cooking Time: 25 Minutes

Servings: 2

Ingredients:

- 2 teaspoons avocado oil
- 6 ounces grass-fed hanger steak, pat dried

- Salt to taste
- 2 cups grated cauliflower
- 2 slices bacon, minced
- 2 pasture raised eggs
- 1 avocado, peeled, pitted, chopped
- 2 cups mixed greens
- 2 cups arugula

For cilantro lime vinaigrette:

- 2 teaspoons MCT oil or Brain octane oil
- 4 tablespoons olive oil
- 1 teaspoon lime juice
- ½ teaspoon sea salt
- 2 teaspoons apple cider vinegar
- ½ cup chopped cilantro

Directions:

1. To make bacon cauliflower rice: Add bacon into a pan and cook until soft and done.
2. Stir in cauliflower rice and sauté for 4 minutes. Turn off the heat.
3. Season a generous amount of salt on either side of the steak.
4. Place a skillet over medium flame. Add the oil, and once it's heated, add the steak and cook until the brown underneath. Turn sides and cook the other side for 3–4 minutes.

5. Remove steak from the pan and place it on the cutting board.

6. When cool enough to handle, cut the steak into slices against the grain.

7. To cook eggs: Meanwhile, place a pot of water to boil. Lower the eggs into the boiling water and cook for 7 minutes.

8. Drain and immerse in plain water for a few minutes. Peel the eggs. Cut into quarters.

9. For cilantro lime dressing: Add all ingredients in a blender. Blend for about a minute or until it's all well combined.

10. Add bacon cauliflower rice, eggs, avocado, steak, and greens into a bowl and toss well.

11. Serve.

Nutrition:

- Calories: 767
- Fat: 63 g
- Total Carbohydrate: 18 g
- Digestible carbohydrate: 8 g
- Edible fibers: 10 g
- Protein: 35 g

36. Crispy Sesame Beef

Preparation Time: 5 Minutes

Cooking Time: 30 Minutes

Servings: 8

Ingredients:

- 2 medium daikon radishes (about 1.5 pound in all)
- 2 tablespoons coconut flour
- 2 tablespoons coconut oil
- 2 teaspoons sesame oil
- 3 tablespoons rice vinegar
- 1 teaspoon red pepper flakes
- 1 medium jalapeno pepper, thinly sliced
- 1 medium red pepper, sliced into thin strips
- 2 medium green onions, chopped
- 2 teaspoons ginger, minced
- 2 garlic cloves, minced
- 2 pounds rib-eye steak, sliced into ¼" strips
- 1 teaspoon guar gum
- ½ cup soy sauce or tamari

- 2 teaspoons oyster sauce
- 2 teaspoons Sriracha
- 2 tablespoons sesame seeds, toasted
- 10 drops Liquid Stevia (optional)
- Oil for frying, as required

Directions:

1. Make noodles of the daikon radish using a spiralizer or julienne peeler.
2. Soak the noodles in a bowl of cold water for about 20–25 minutes. Drain in a colander.
3. Place a large frying pan or wok over high flame. Add the oil, and once it's heated add ginger, garlic, and red pepper. Sauté until it gets fragrant. Add sesame seeds and sauté for a couple of minutes.
4. Add soy sauce, oyster sauce, sesame oil, vinegar, Sriracha, and stevia. Mix well and let it cook for a couple of minutes. Remove from heat.
5. Meanwhile, place a deep pan over medium flame. Pour enough oil into the pan so that it covers at least an inch in height from the bottom of the pan.
6. When the temperature of the oil is nearly 325ºF, add beef strips in batches and cook until brown all over.
7. Remove the strips and place them on paper towels.
8. Place the wok over medium flame. Add the crispy beef strips and mixture of sauces and cook for a couple of minutes.
9. To serve: Divide equally the daikon noodles and place on individual serving plates. Top with a few crispy beef strips along with sauce and serve.

Nutrition:

- Calories: 412

- Fat: 31.3 g
- Total Carbohydrate: 8.8 g
- Digestible carbohydrate: 5 g
- Edible fibers: 3.8 g
- Protein: 24.5 g

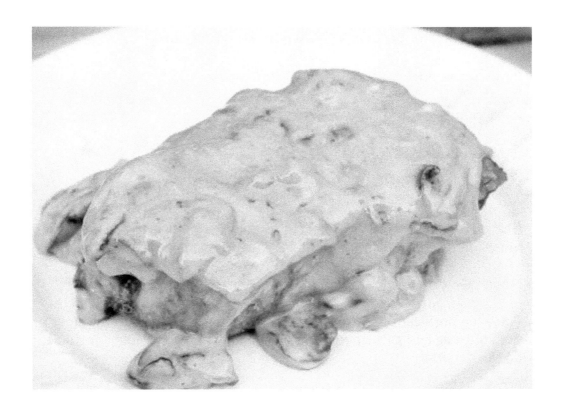

37. Fat Bomb Pork Chops

Preparation Time: 5 Minutes

Cooking Time: 30 Minutes

Servings: 6

Ingredients:

- 2 medium yellow onions, sliced
- 1 cup oil

- 2 teaspoons garlic powder
- 2 cups keto-friendly mayonnaise
- 2 packages (8 ounces each) brown mushrooms, sliced
- 6 medium boneless pork chops
- 2 teaspoons ground nutmeg
- 2 tablespoons balsamic vinegar

Directions:

1. Heat a large skillet over low heat. Add the oil, and once it's heated, add onions and mushrooms and cook until onions are translucent.
2. Move the vegetables to one of the sides of the skillet.
3. Place the pork chops in the center of the skillet. Season both the sides of the pork with nutmeg and garlic powder. Cook until the pork is cooked inside and brown on the outside.
4. Remove pork and place it on a plate.
5. Move the onion and mushrooms to the center of the pan. Add mayonnaise and vinegar and stir until well combined. If you find the sauce very thick, add a little water or broth and stir.
6. Spoon the sauce over the chops and serve.

Nutrition:

- Calories: 1121
- Fat: 104 g
- Total Carbohydrate: 9 g
- Digestible carbohydrate: 8 g

- Edible fibers: 1 g
- Protein: 35 g

38. Italian Sausage Stuffed Mushrooms

Preparation Time: 5 Minutes

Cooking Time: 20 Minutes

Servings: 8

Ingredients:

- 8 Jumbo Portobello mushroom caps, remove stems
- 2 cups shredded Pepper Jack cheese
- ½ cup chopped fresh basil
- Salt to taste
- 2 pounds Italian sausage
- 3 cups keto-friendly marinara sauce
- 4 garlic cloves, minced
- Pepper to taste

Directions:

1. Place the mushroom caps on a lined baking sheet, with the stem part facing up.
2. Place the baking sheet in a preheated oven and bake at 375ºF for about 15 to 20 minutes or until slightly soft.
3. In the meantime, place a skillet over medium-high flame. Place sausage in the pan and cook until brown. Break it simultaneously as it cooks.
4. Lower the heat to medium flame. Stir in the garlic and cook until aromatic.

5. Add the remaining ingredients, except cheese and mix well. Discard any cooked liquid from the mushrooms.

6. Stuff the sausage mixture into the mushroom caps. Sprinkle cheese on top.

7. Broil in an oven until cheese melts and is browned as per your desire.

Nutrition:

- Calories: 578
- Fat: 47 g
- Total Carbohydrate: 12 g
- Digestible carbohydrate: 10 g
- Edible fibers: 2 g
- Protein: 26 g

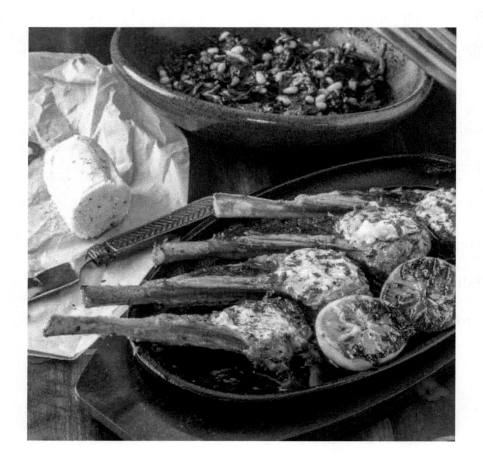

39. Lamb Chops with Herb Butter

Preparation Time: 5 Minutes

Cooking Time: 10 Minutes

Servings: 2

Ingredients:

- 4 lamb chops, at room temperature

- ½ tablespoon olive oil
- ½ tablespoon butter
- Salt to taste
- Pepper to taste
- Lemon wedges, to serve
- 2 ounces herb butter, to serve

Directions:

1. Sprinkle salt and pepper over the lamb chops.
2. Place a skillet over medium flame. Heat oil and butter in the skillet and when butter melts, add lamb chops and cook to the desired doneness.
3. Remove from the pan and place on individual serving plates. Top with butter and serve with lemon wedges.

Nutrition:

- Calories: 723
- Fat: 62 g
- Total Carbohydrate: 0.3 g
- Digestible carbohydrate: 0.3 g
- Edible fibers: 0 g
- Protein: 43 g

40. Lamb Burgers

Preparation Time: 5 Minutes

Cooking Time: 15 Minutes

Servings: 5

Ingredients:

For lamb and halloumi burgers:

- 1 pound ground lamb
- 1 egg
- ½ tablespoons finely chopped parsley
- Salt to taste
- Pepper to taste
- 4.5 ounces halloumi cheese, grated
- 1 teaspoon ground cumin
- ½ teaspoon finely chopped rosemary

For cucumber cream:

- 4 ounces sour cream
- ½ teaspoon ground cumin
- Pepper to taste
- Salt to taste

- 1.75 ounces cucumber, deseeded, finely diced

Directions:

1. For the burgers: Add ground lamb, egg, parsley, seasonings, cheese, cumin, and rosemary into a bowl and mix well.

2. Make 5 equal portions of the lamb mixture and shape into patties.

3. Keep a grill pan over medium-high flame. When the pan heats, cook the burgers in batches for 5 to 8 minutes or to the desired doneness. You can also grill the burgers on a preheated grill.

4. Meanwhile, add all ingredients for cucumber cream into a bowl and mix well.

5. Serve burgers with cucumber cream.

Nutrition:

- Calories: 397
- Fat: 33 g
- Total Carbohydrate: 1 g
- Digestible carbohydrate: 1 g
- Edible fibers: 0 g
- Protein: 22 g

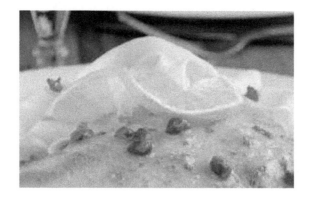

41. Fish in Lemon Butter Caper Sauce

Preparation Time: 5 Minutes

Cooking Time: 5 Minutes

Servings: 4

Ingredients:

- 1.1 pounds fish fillets
- 1-ounce capers
- 2 garlic cloves, minced
- tablespoons olive oil
- Salt to taste
- Pepper to taste
- 5.6 ounces butter

- 1 medium onion, chopped
- 1 tablespoon chopped parsley
- Lemon juice to drizzle

Directions:

1. Place a nonstick pan with oil over medium flame.
2. Place fish in the pan and sprinkle salt and pepper over it. Cook until the fish is cooked.
3. Transfer the fish into a bowl.
4. Place onions in the same pan and cook until translucent.
5. Stir in a little of the butter and let it melt. Add garlic and cook until fragrant.
6. Stir in the capers. Break it with a spatula. Add a little more butter and parsley and stir until butter melts. Remove from heat.
7. Add remaining butter and lemon juice and stir.
8. Spoon the sauce over the fish and serve.

Nutrition:

- Calories: 392
- Fat: 32 g
- Total Carbohydrate: 9 g
- Digestible carbohydrate: 7 g
- Edible fibers: 2 g
- Protein: 18 g

42. Creamy Garlic Shrimp

Preparation Time: 5 Minutes

Cooking Time: 10 Minutes

Servings: 8

Ingredients:

- 2 tablespoons olive oil
- Salt to taste
- Pepper to taste
- 12 garlic cloves, minced
- 3 cups reduced fat cream
- ¼ cup chopped parsley
- 2 pounds shrimp
- 4 tablespoons unsalted butter
- 1 cup chicken broth
- 1 cup freshly grated parmesan cheese

Directions:

1. Place a large skillet with oil over medium-high flame and heat the oil.
2. Sprinkle salt and pepper over the shrimp and place in the skillet. Cook for a couple of minutes. Turn over the shrimp and cook for a couple of minutes or until pink. Remove the shrimp from the pan and place in a bowl.

3. Add butter into the skillet. When butter melts, add garlic and stir-fry for a few seconds until aromatic.

4. Stir in the broth and scrape the bottom of the pan using the spatula to loosen any brown bits that may be stuck.

5. Once it starts to boil, lower the heat to medium-low. Stir in the cream. Add salt and pepper to taste.

6. When it begins to bubble, add parmesan cheese and let it cook for a minute.

7. Add shrimp and parsley and stir until shrimp is well coated with the sauce. Turn off the heat.

8. Serve over keto-friendly pasta or cauliflower rice.

Nutrition:

- Calories: 488
- Fat: 44 g
- Total Carbohydrate: 4 g
- Digestible carbohydrate: 4 g
- Edible fibers: 0 g
- Protein: 30 g

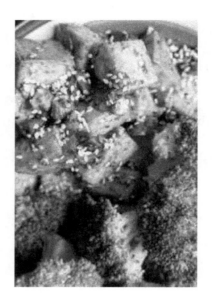

43. Spicy Almond Tofu

Preparation Time: 5 Minutes

Cooking Time: 15 Minutes

Servings: 4

Ingredients:

- 1 teaspoon garlic powder
- ½ cup water
- 4 teaspoons sesame oil
- 8 tablespoons green chili sauce

- 1 teaspoon Himalayan pink salt or more to taste
- 1 teaspoon paprika
- 1 teaspoon onion powder
- 8 tablespoons liquid aminos
- ½ teaspoon chili flakes
- 4 packages firm tofu or extra-firm tofu, pressed of excess moisture, cubed
- 4 tablespoons coconut oil
- 4 tablespoons sesame seeds, divided
- 1 teaspoon pepper to taste
- ½ cup sliced almonds

Directions:

1. Heat a skillet with coconut oil over medium flame. Once the oil gets heated, add tofu and cook until golden brown on all the sides and is crisp.
2. Add almonds and cook for a couple of minutes. Retain ½ tablespoon sesame seeds and sesame oil and add the rest of the ingredients. Cook until all the liquid in the pan is absorbed.
3. Serving over steamed broccoli or any other steamed vegetables is a good option. Drizzle sesame oil over tofu. Sprinkle remaining sesame seeds on top and serve.

Nutrition:

- Calories: 400
- Fat: 29 g
- Total Carbohydrate: 10 g
- Digestible carbohydrate: 5 g

- Edible fibers: 5 g
- Protein: 24 g

44. Vegan Dinner Bowl

Preparation Time: 5 Minutes

Cooking Time: 30 Minutes

Servings: 2

Ingredients:

For baked tofu:

- ½ package firm tofu, pressed of excess moisture
- ½ teaspoon garlic powder
- Pepper to taste
- 1 tablespoon soy sauce or tamari
- ½ tablespoon arrowroot powder

For almond butter sauce:

- 2 tablespoons almond butter or sunflower seed butter
- ½ tablespoon unseasoned rice wine vinegar
- 2 tablespoons unsweetened almond or coconut milk
- Salt to taste
- Pepper to taste
- 1 tablespoon soy sauce or tamari
- 1 teaspoon sriracha sauce

- 5 drops liquid stevia

For cabbage rice:

- ¼ cup chopped green onions
- ½ small green cabbage, cut into chunks
- 2 garlic cloves, minced
- ½ teaspoon coconut oil
- ¼ cup chopped cilantro

For bowl:

- 1 small avocado, peeled, pitted, chopped
- 2 cups chopped kale, steamed
- 2 cups broccoli florets, steamed

Directions:

1. Add all ingredients for baked tofu into a bowl and toss well. Place on a lined baking sheet and spread it evenly.

2. Place the baking sheet in a preheated oven and bake at 375ºF for about 15 to 20 minutes or until brown.

3. To make cabbage rice: Place cabbage in the food processor bowl and process until it is rice-like in texture.

4. Place a skillet over high flame. Add cabbage and remaining ingredients for cabbage rice and mix well. Do not stir for about 2–3 minutes. Stir again. Repeat this a few times until the cabbage is slightly brown.

5. For almond butter sauce: Add almond butter, vinegar, milk, pepper, soy sauce, salt, sriracha, and stevia into a bowl and whisk well.

6. To make bowls: Divide cabbage rice among 2 bowls. Layer with kale and broccoli, followed by avocado and tofu. Drizzle sauce on top and serve.

Nutrition:

- Calories: 423
- Fat: 27 g
- Total Carbohydrate: 30 g
- Digestible carbohydrate: 16 g
- Edible fibers: 14 g
- Protein: 23 g

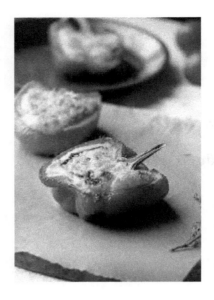

45. Cheese Quiche Stuffed Peppers

Preparation Time: 5 Minutes

Cooking Time: 45 Minutes

Servings: 2

Ingredients:

- 1 medium bell pepper, halved lengthwise, deseeded
- ¼ cup ricotta cheese
- ¼ cup grated parmesan cheese + 1 tablespoon to garnish
- 1/8 teaspoon dried parsley
- 2 large eggs

- ¼ cup shredded mozzarella cheese
- ½ teaspoon garlic powder
- A handful baby spinach leaves, chopped

Directions:

1. Add eggs, parsley, garlic powder, parmesan cheese, mozzarella cheese, and ricotta cheese into the food processor bowl and process until well combined.
2. Fill this mixture into the bell pepper halves. Do not fill up to the top.
3. Place spinach leaves on top and press the leaves lightly into the filling.
4. Place a sheet of foil on top of the bell pepper halves.
5. Place the baking sheet in a preheated oven and bake at 375ºF for about 30 to 40 minutes or until the eggs are cooked.
6. Uncover and broil for a couple of minutes until light brown on top.

Nutrition:

- Calories: 245.5
- Fat: 16.28 g
- Total Carbohydrate: 7.1 g
- Digestible carbohydrate: 5.97 g
- Edible fibers: 1.13 g
- Protein: 17.84 g

Chapter 4: Vegan Keto Recipes

46. P. F. Chang's® Spicy Green Beans

Preparation Time: 10 Minutes

Cooking Time: 10 Minutes

Servings: 4

Ingredients:

- 1 pound of green beans, rinsed and trimmed
- 2 tablespoons of fresh ginger, grated
- 2 tablespoons of garlic, minced
- 2 tablespoons of cooking oil
- ¼ cup of water

Sauce:

- 2 tablespoons of soy sauce
- 1 tablespoon of rice vinegar
- 2 teaspoons of sugar
- 2 tablespoons of Szechuan peppercorn

Directions:

1. Combine all the sauce ingredients in a bowl.

2. Bring some water to a boil and add the green beans.

3. Cook for 3 to 5 minutes, or until crispy.

4. Sauté the garlic and ginger in the oil.

5. When the mixture becomes aromatic, add in the green beans and cook for 2 to 3 minutes, or until soft.

6. Add in the sauce and continue stirring the beans.

7. Serve.

Nutrition:

- Calories: 117.4 kcal
- Fat: 7.1 g
- Carbs: 12.4g
- Protein: 3.3g

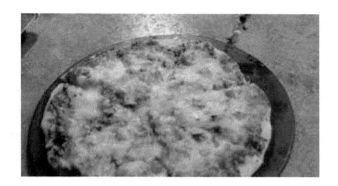

47. Applebee® Veggie Patch Pizza

Preparation Time: 5 Minutes

Cooking Time: 10 Minutes

Servings: 1

Ingredients:

- 1 (10-inch) flour tortilla
- 1 teaspoon olive oil
- ½ cup hot spinach and artichoke dip
- ¼ cup tomatoes, diced
- ½ cup mushrooms, sliced
- Salt and pepper to taste
- ¼ teaspoon garlic powder

- ½ teaspoon Italian seasoning
- ½ cup mozzarella cheese, shredded
- 1 tablespoon Parmesan/Romano cheese, shredded

Directions:

1. Preheat the oven to 350°F.
2. If you are using a pizza stone, place it in the oven to get hot. (Even though you are using a tortilla for the crust, the pizza stone will help make it crispy.)
3. With a pastry brush, brush the tortilla on both sides with olive oil.
4. Place the tortilla on the pizza stone, and top it with the spinach and artichoke dip, diced tomatoes, and mushrooms.
5. Sprinkle the spices on the top of the tomatoes and mushrooms, and top with the cheeses. Bake for approximately 10 minutes or until the cheese is melted and bubbly.

Nutrition:

- Calories: 151kcal
- Fat: 9g
- Carbs: 10.3g
- Protein: 7.4g

48. Applebee® Vegetable Medley

Preparation Time: 15 Minutes

Cooking Time: 10 Minutes

Servings: 4

Ingredients:

- ½ pound of cold, fresh zucchini, sliced in half moons
- ½ pound of cold, fresh yellow squash, sliced in half moons
- ¼ pound of cold red pepper, julienned in strips ¼-inch thick
- ¼ pound of cold carrots, cut in ¼-inch strips a few inches long
- ¼ pound of cold red onions, thinly sliced
- 1 cold, small corn cob, cut crosswise in 1" segments
- 3 tablespoons of cold butter or margarine
- 1 teaspoon of salt
- 1 teaspoon of sugar
- ½ teaspoon of granulated garlic
- 1 teaspoon of Worcestershire sauce
- 1 teaspoon of soy sauce
- 2 teaspoons of fresh or dried parsley

Directions:

1. Wash, peel, and cut your vegetables as appropriate.
2. In a saucepan, heat the butter over medium-high heat.
3. Once it is hot, add the salt, sugar, and garlic.
4. Add the carrots, squash, and zucchini, and when they start to soften, add the rest of the vegetables and cook for a couple of minutes.
5. Add the Worcestershire sauce, soy sauce and parsley.
6. Stir to combine and coat the vegetables.
7. When all the vegetables are cooked to your preference, serve.

Nutrition:

- Calories: 170 kcal
- Fat: 2g
- Carbs: 18g
- Protein: 15g

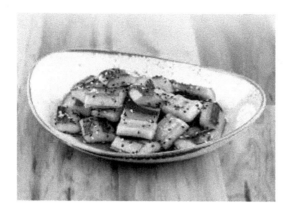

49. PF Chang's® Shanghai Cucumbers

Preparation Time: 5 Minutes

Cooking Time: 0 Minutes

Servings: 4

Ingredients:

- 2 English cucumbers, peeled and chopped
- 3 tablespoons of soy sauce
- ½ teaspoon of sesame oil
- 1 teaspoon of white vinegar
- Sprinkle of toasted sesame seeds

Directions:

1. Stir together the soy sauce, sesame oil and vinegar in a serving dish.

2. Add the cucumbers and toss to coat.

3. Sprinkle with the sesame seeds.

Nutrition:

- Calories: 70 kcal
- Fat: 3g
- Carbs: 7g
- Protein: 4g

50. Chili® Black Bean

Preparation Time: 5 Minutes

Cooking Time: 25 Minutes

Servings: 6

Ingredients:

- 2 cans (15.5 ounces each) of black beans
- ½ teaspoon of sugar
- 1 teaspoon of ground cumin
- 1 teaspoon of chili powder
- ½ teaspoon of garlic powder
- 2 tablespoons of red onion, diced finely
- ½ teaspoon of fresh cilantro, minced (optional)
- ½ cup of water
- Salt and black pepper to taste
- Pico de Gallo and or sour cream for garnish (optional)

Directions:

1. Combine the beans, sugar, cumin, chili powder, garlic, onion, cilantro (if using), and water in a saucepan and mix well.
2. Over medium-low heat, let the bean mixture simmer for about 20–25 minutes. Season with salt and pepper to taste.
3. Remove the beans from heat and transfer to serving bowls.

4. Garnish with Pico de Gallo and a dollop of sour cream, if desired.

Nutrition:

- Calories: 143.8
- Fat: 0.7g
- Carbs: 25.9g
- Protein: 9.5.2g

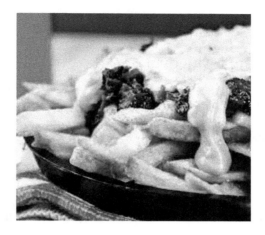

51. In "N" Out® Animal Style Fries

Preparation Time: 10 Minutes

Cooking Time: 30 Minutes

Servings: 8

Ingredients:

- 32 ounces of frozen French fries
- 2 cups of cheddar cheese, shredded
- 1 large onion, diced
- 2 tablespoons of raw sugar
- 2 tablespoons of olive oil
- 1 ½ cups of mayonnaise

- ¾ cup of ketchup
- ¼ cup of sweet relish
- 1 ½ teaspoons of white sugar
- 1 ½ teaspoons of apple cider vinegar
- ½ teaspoon of salt
- ½ teaspoon of black pepper

Directions:

1. Preheat oven to 350°F and place the oven grill in the middle position.
2. Place fries on a large baking sheet and bake in the oven according to package's directions.
3. In the meantime, warm the olive oil in a large non-stick skillet over medium heat.
4. Add the onions and sauté for about 2 minutes until fragrant and soft.
5. Add raw sugar and continue cooking until the onions caramelize.
6. Remove from heat and set aside.
7. Add the mayonnaise, ketchup, relish, white sugar, salt, and black pepper to a bowl and mix until well combined. Set aside.
8. Once the fries are cooked, remove from heat and set the oven to broil.
9. Sprinkle with the cheddar cheese over the fries and place under the broiler until the cheese melts, about 2–3 minutes. Add the cheese fries to serving bowls or plates. Add some caramelized onions on top and smother with mayonnaise sauce.
10. Serve immediately.

Nutrition:

- Calories: 750 kcal

- Fat: 42g
- Carbs: 54g
- Protein: 19g

52. KFC® Coleslaw

Preparation Time: 15 Minutes

Cooking Time: 0 Minutes

Servings: 10

Ingredients:

- 8 cups of cabbage, finely diced
- ¼ cup of carrot, finely diced
- 2 tablespoons of onions, minced
- 1/3 cup of granulated sugar
- ½ teaspoon of salt
- 1/8 teaspoon of pepper
- ¼ cup of milk
- ½ cup of mayonnaise
- ¼ cup of buttermilk
- 1½ tablespoons of white vinegar
- 2½ tablespoons of lemon juice

Directions:

1. Mix the cabbage, carrot, and onions in a bowl.
2. Place the rest of the ingredients in a blender or food processor and blend until smooth.

3. Pour the sauce over the cabbage mixture.

4. Place in the refrigerator for several hours before serving.

Nutrition:

- Calories: 170 kcal
- Fat: 12g
- Carbs: 14g
- Protein: 4g

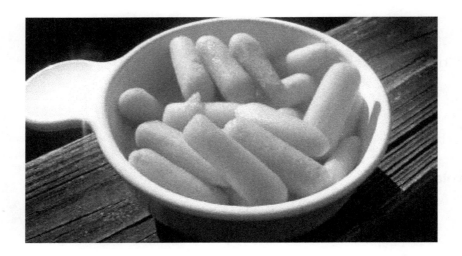

53. Cracker Barrel® Baby Carrot

Preparation Time: 5 Minutes

Cooking Time: 45 Minutes

Servings: 6

Ingredients:

- 1 teaspoon of bacon grease, melted
- 2 pounds of fresh baby carrots
- Some water
- 1 teaspoon of salt
- ¼ cup of brown sugar
- ¼ cup of butter, melted

- ¼ cup of honey

Directions:

1. Heat the bacon grease in a pot.
2. Place the carrots in the grease and sauté for 10 seconds.
3. Cover the carrots with water and add the salt.
4. Bring the entire mixture to a boil over medium heat, then reduce the heat to low and allow it to simmer for another 30 to 45 minutes.
5. By this time, the carrots should be half cooked.
6. Remove half the water from the pot and add the rest of the ingredients.
7. Keep cooking until the carrots become tender.
8. Transfer to a bowl and serve.

Nutrition:

- Calories: 80 kcal
- Fat: 1g
- Carbs: 18g
- Protein: 1g

54. Olive Garden® Gnocchi with Spicy Tomato and Wine Sauce

Preparation Time: 10 Minutes

Cooking Time: 40 Minutes

Servings: 4

Ingredients:

Sauce:

- 2 tablespoons of extra virgin olive oil
- 6 fresh garlic cloves
- ½ teaspoon of chili flakes
- 1 cup of dry white wine
- 1 cup of chicken broth
- 2 cans (14.5 ounces each) of tomatoes
- ¼ cup of fresh basil, chopped
- ¼ cup of sweet creamy butter, cut into 1-inch cubes, chilled
- ½ cup of parmesan cheese, freshly grated

Pasta:

- 1 pound of gnocchi
- Salt, to taste
- Black pepper, freshly crushed, to taste

Directions:

1. Place the olive oil, garlic, and chili flakes in a cold pan and cook over medium heat.
2. When the garlic starts turning golden brown, add the wine and broth and bring the mixture to a simmer.
3. After about 10 minutes, the broth should be halved.
4. When that happens, add in the tomatoes and basil, and then let the sauce continue simmering for another 30 minutes.
5. Once the sauce has thickened, set it aside to cool for 3 minutes.
6. After 3 minutes, place the sauce in a blender, and add the butter and parmesan.
7. Purée everything together and set aside.
8. Prepare the pasta by boiling the gnocchi in a large pot.
9. When it is cooked, strain the pasta and mix with the sauce.
10. Transfer everything to a plate and serve.

Nutrition:

- Calories: 285.8 kcal
- Fat: 18.9g
- Carbs: 12.1g
- Protein: 8.4g

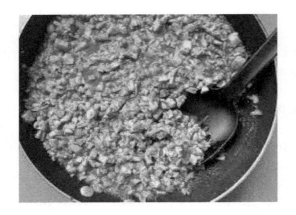

55. Chipotle® Sofritas

Preparation Time: 10 Minutes

Cooking Time: 25 Minutes

Servings: 4

Ingredients:

Mexican Spice Mix:

- ½ teaspoon of dried oregano leaves
- 2 teaspoons of ancho chili powder, ground
- 1 teaspoon of cumin, ground
- ½ teaspoon of coriander, ground
- ½ teaspoon of kosher salt

Sofritas:

- 1 tablespoon of avocado or olive oil
- ½ medium onion, diced
- 2 garlic cloves, minced
- 1 teaspoon of chipotle chili in adobo sauce, minced
- 1 tablespoon of mild Hatch chili, diced
- 1 tablespoon of Mexican Spice Mix
- 2 tablespoons of tomato paste
- 1 package (16 ounces) of organic extra firm tofu, drained, dried, crumbled
- 1 cup of your favorite Mexican beer
- Salt and black pepper to taste
- Tortillas and lime wedges for garnish

Directions:

1. Place all the Mexican Spice Mix ingredients in a container or plastic bag and shake to mix.
2. Sauté the onion and garlic in oil over medium heat for 5 minutes.
3. Mix in both the chilies and the spice mix and sauté for another minute.
4. Pour in the tomato paste and cook for a minute.
5. Add the rest of the ingredients and cook for 5 more minutes.
6. Taste and adjust seasoning with salt and pepper if required.
7. Remove the mixture from heat, transfer to a bowl, and then serve with tortillas and thin lime wedges.

Nutrition:

- Calories: 470 kcal
- Fat: 19g
- Carbs: 59g
- Protein: 16g
- Sodium: 1160mg

56. Melting Pot® Green Goddess Dip

Preparation Time: 5 Minutes

Cooking Time: 5 Minutes

Servings: 12

Ingredients:

- 8 ounces of cheese, sliced
- 1/2 cup of milk
- 1/4 cup of cream
- 2 tbsp. of onion
- 2 tbsp. of parsley
- 2 tbsp. of chives

Directions:

1. Microwave cheese and milk in a healthy container for 2–4 minutes, whisking after each minute, before adding the cream cheese. Melt and mix smoothly.
2. Stir in sour cream, cabbage, chives, and parsley.
3. Refrigerate before serving and enjoy!

Nutrition:

- Calories: 85 kcal
- Fat: 7.8g
- Carbs: 1.6g

- Protein: 1.6g

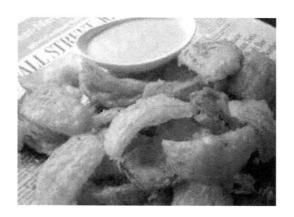

57. Applebee's Onion Peels

Preparation Time: 5 Minutes

Cooking Time: 25 Minutes

Servings: 6

Ingredients:

Horseradish dipping sauce:

- 1/2 cup of mayonnaise
- 1 tbsp. of prepared horseradish
- 2 tsp. of white vinegar
- 1 tsp. of water
- 1 tsp. of paprika
- 1 tsp. of ketchup

- 1/4 tsp. of black pepper
- 1/8 tsp. of dried oregano
- 1/8 tsp. of cayenne
- 1/4 tsp. of garlic powder
- 1/4 tsp. of onion powder

Batter:

- 5–6 cups of shortening
- 1 large onion
- 1/2 cup of all-purpose flour
- 1/2 cup of Progresso Plain Bread Crumbs
- 1/2 tsp. of salt
- 1/2 tsp. of black pepper
- 1 1/2 cups of milk

Directions:

1. Make horseradish dipping sauce, mixing ingredients with a whisk in a medium cup.
2. Then blend the sauce until smooth, cover, and chill.
3. Heat the shortening on a deep fryer to 350°F.
4. Slice the end of the stem and the end of the root off the onion, then cut through the onion, slice it in half with the onion lying on a flat side. Slice each half 4 to 5 times more to make onion wedges in a spoken fashion.
5. Separate pieces of an onion.

6. Mix all the dry ingredients into a medium bowl to make batter.

7. Whisk in the milk until smooth batter, then let the batter sit for 5 minutes. It should grow thicker.

8. Then again whisk the batter.

9. Dip pieces of onion in the batter, when the oil is hot, let some of the batter drip off, and then carefully drop the piece of coated onion into the hot oil. Repeat for 1 to 2 minutes, or until light brown, frying 8 to 12 at a time. Drain onto a towel rack or notebook.

10. Repeat until the onion is removed, stack the newer lots on top of the old lots to keep them dry.

11. Serve fried onion slices on a plate or in a paper-coated basket with horseradish dipping sauce on the side when they are all done.

Nutrition:

- Calories: 234 kcal

- Fat: 14g

- Carb: 22g

- Protein: 5g

58. McDonald's® Hash Browns

Preparation Time: 5 Minutes

Cooking Time: 15 Minutes

Servings: 6

Ingredients:

- 4 Potatoes
- Ice cold water
- 2 tbsp. of Butter
- 2 tbsp. of Rice flour
- Red chili powder to test
- 1 tsp. of Salt or to taste
- 1 tsp. of Onion powder
- 1 tsp. of Black pepper powder
- 1 tsp. of Corn flour
- 3 tbsp. of Cheddar cheese, grated
- Oil for frying

Directions:

1. Cut potatoes with a grater.
2. Remove rubbed potatoes in ice cold water for 10 minutes, then drain and squeeze with muslin cloth and set aside full.

3. Add butter and melt in wok, add the grated and squeeze potatoes, mix well and cook on medium flame for 4–5 minutes and allow to cool.

4. Add rice flour, red chili powder, salt, ionic powder, black pepper powder, corn flour and cheddar cheese, blend well and leave to stand for 5 minutes.

5. Grease the oil on your palms, take a mixture and make an oval shape of similar size.

6. Heat oil and cook in a frying pan until golden brown.

Nutrition:

- Calories: 260 kcal
- Fat: 10g
- Carbs: 26g
- Protein: 2g

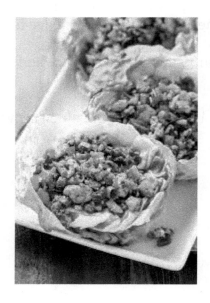

59. P. F. Chang's® Vegetarian Lettuce Wraps

Preparation Time: 10 Minutes

Cooking Time: 10 Minutes

Servings: 6

Ingredients:

- 13 ounces of firm tofu
- 2 tbsp. of avocado oil
- 1 cups of mushrooms
- 1/2 cup of onions

- 1 (7 ounces) can of sliced water chestnuts
- 4 ounces of bamboo shoots chopped
- 3 garlic cloves
- 1/2 carrot, shredded
- 1 head of lettuce
- 1 teaspoon of sesame seeds
- 1/4 cup of cilantro leaves

For Sauce:

- 2 tbsp. of vegetarian mushroom oyster sauce
- 2 tbsp. of hoisin sauce
- 1 tbsp. of low sodium soy sauce
- 1 tbsp. of wine vinegar
- 2 stalks of chopped scallions
- 1 tbsp. of sesame oil

Directions:

1. Heat over high heat a non-stick pan and add the oil.
2. Crumble the tofu into the oven, so that it looks like ground tofu.
3. Sauté the tofu over high heat until the tofu turns a light brown, golden color.
4. Low to medium heat. Remove mushrooms, onions, water chestnuts, garlic and bamboo shoots.
5. Sauté the onions for 1–2 minutes before they start softening.

6. Place the ingredients for the sauce into the pan and sauté for another 1–2 minutes.

7. Season with salt and pepper.

8. Place two lettuce leaves on top and spoon the tofu filling in the middle.

9. Sprinkle on sesame seeds and garnish with shredded carrots and cilantro leaves.

Nutrition:

- Calories: 610 kcal
- Fat: 36g
- Carbs: 39g
- Protein: 25g

60. Houston® Veggie Burger

Preparation Time: 15 Minutes

Cooking Time: 10 Minutes

Servings: 4

Ingredients:

- 1 can of black beans
- 1 tsp. of olive oil
- ¼ cup of onion, chopped
- 1 garlic clove
- 1 tsp. of smoked paprika
- 1 tsp. of cumin
- ½ tsp. of chili powder
- 1 tsp. of kosher salt
- Black pepper, to taste
- ¼ cup of BBQ sauce
- 1 tbsp. of molasses
- ¼ cup of oats
- 1 ¼ cup of cooked brown rice
- 2 tbsp. of canned beets, finely chopped

- 1 tbsp. of beet juice
- 1 egg
- 4 whole wheat hamburger buns

Directions:

1. The beans are added to a large mixing bowl.
2. Gently pat dry beans, with a towel of paper.
3. Mash beans until smooth and pasty using the rear side of a fork or potato masher.
4. Heat a small skillet. Add the olive oil, onion and garlic when hot.
5. Sauté with the beans for 3 minutes, then move to the pot.
6. Add the paprika, cumin, chili powder, salt and pepper in a small bowl.
7. Mix and transfer to the wide bowl until mixed.
8. Mix the BBQ sauce and molasses with the same small pot, until completely mixed.
9. Add 3 spoonful of the mixture to the large bowl and set the rest aside for cooking.
10. Process oats in a food processor equipped with a metal blade until finely finished.
11. Add the oats and the beans, vegetables, and sauce to the large cup.
12. Add the rice, beets, beet juice and egg; and mix everything until cool.
13. Form the mixture into 4 patties, around 5 1/2 ounces each, using your hands.
14. Place the patties on plate for freezer and freeze for 30 minutes.
15. Alternatively, you can place them 2 hours or more in the refrigerator.
16. Size a medium-heat large flat skillet.
17. Spray with butter, and move patties to the skillet using a spatula.

18. Cook the patties for 5 minutes, flip thoroughly with the spatula, baste with the remaining sauce and cook for another 5 minutes.

19. Add cheese, if used, within the last 2 minutes.

20. Place each patty on a bun with the spatula, and top with the appropriate toppings.

Nutrition:

- Calories: 302 kcal
- Fat: 4g
- Carbs: 56g
- Protein: 11g

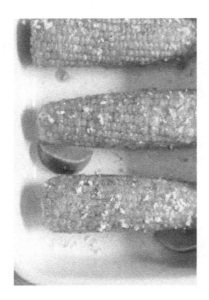

61. Disneyland® Chili Lime Corn on the Cob

Preparation Time: 10 Minutes

Cooking Time: 5 Minutes

Servings: 4

Ingredients:

- 5 ears of sweet corn
- 1/4 cup of butter
- 1 tsp. of chili powder
- 2 tbsp. of lime juice

- 1 Lime
- 1/4 cup of Cotija cheese, for topping

Directions:

1. Fill a (large) stockpot with heat and water to boil.
2. Attach the corn and cook for 6–7 minutes, until warm.
3. Add butter, chili powder and lime juice in a (shallow) dish while the corn is cooking.
4. Remove that corn from stockpot and roll it in a mixture of butter.
5. Top with Cotija cheese and lime zest (optional) and serve dry.

Nutrition:

- Calories: 422 kcal
- Fat: 46g
- Carbs: 2g
- Protein: 1g

62. Tony Roma® Maple Sweet Potatoes

Preparation Time: 10 Minutes

Cooking Time: 30 Minutes

Servings: 4

Ingredients:

- 1 sweet potato
- 1 tbsp. of butter
- 1/4 of an onion, chopped
- 3 tbsp. of finely chopped pecans
- 3 tbsp. of maple syrup
- ¼ tsp. of cinnamon

Directions:

1. Bake the sweet potato in the oven.
2. This will almost bake the potato all the way through, while still letting it slice firm enough when cool.
3. Take the potato out of the oven and let it cool, to be able to handle it.
4. Once cooled, remove the skin and slice to cubes.
5. Melt the butter in a large skillet.
6. Sauté the onion and pecans for a few minutes, or until the onion starts browning.
7. Add the sweet potato, maple syrup and cubed potato.

8. Sauté for 4 to 5 minutes, always stirring, or until the pieces of sweet potatoes are warm and tender.

9. Take out in the sheet and serve!

Nutrition:

- Calories: 381 kcal
- Fat: 42g
- Carbs: 75g
- Protein: 6g

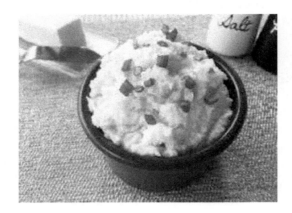

63. Ruby Tuesday® Creamy Mashed Cauliflower

Preparation Time: 15 Minutes

Cooking Time: 45 Minutes

Servings: 4

Ingredients:

- 1 cauliflower
- ¾ cup of water
- 1 tbsp. of cornstarch
- 1/2 cup of heavy cream
- 1 tsp. of granulated sugar
- ¾ tsp. of salt
- ¼ tsp. of white pepper

- 1/8 tsp. of garlic powder
- 1/8 tsp. of onion powder

Directions:

1. Split a cauliflower head into florets that are all about the same size.
2. Steam bits of cauliflower for 15 to 18 minutes, over boiling water, or before tender cauliflower. Drain and throw the cauliflower in a bowl of ice water.
3. When the cauliflower has cooled, put 1/2 cup of water and the florets in a food processor.
4. Puree Mix High speed the cauliflower up to smooth but with
5. A few very small pieces of cauliflower that remain in the Mix just for a bit of texture.
6. Pour the entire pureed cauliflower into a medium Cocktail.
7. Dissolve the cornstarch within remaining cup with water and add cauliflower solution.
8. Stir in the cream, sugar, salt, white pepper and garlic cauliflower powder and onion powder and stir in.
9. Stir the casserole over medium heat, and cook often till thickness.

Nutrition:

- Calories: 136 kcal
- Fat: 8g
- Carbs: 13g
- Protein: 1g

64. P. F. Chang's® Garlic Snap Peas

Preparation Time: 5 Minutes

Cooking Time: 7 Minutes

Servings: 4

Ingredients:

- 2 cups of sugar snap peas
- 2 tsp. of vegetable oil
- 1/8 tsp. of salt
- Black pepper to taste
- 2 garlic cloves

Directions:

1. Prepare the snap peas by separating tips on every single end of the pods.
2. Preheat the oil over a wok or medium skillet on medium to high heat.
3. Sauté the peas in oil with salt and pepper, tossing often for almost 3 minutes, until the peas are cooked, but still crusted.
4. The pods should start to bruise a few dark brown when they're finished, spots grow upon them.
5. Add garlic, toss a little more, then pour the snap peas straight away on a serving dish.
6. If you keep the garlic inside for too long, it could get burnt and bitter, so don't leave it in the hot pan for longer than 10 seconds.

Nutrition:

- Calories: 110 kcal
- Fat: 3.5g
- Carbs: 12g
- Protein: 3g

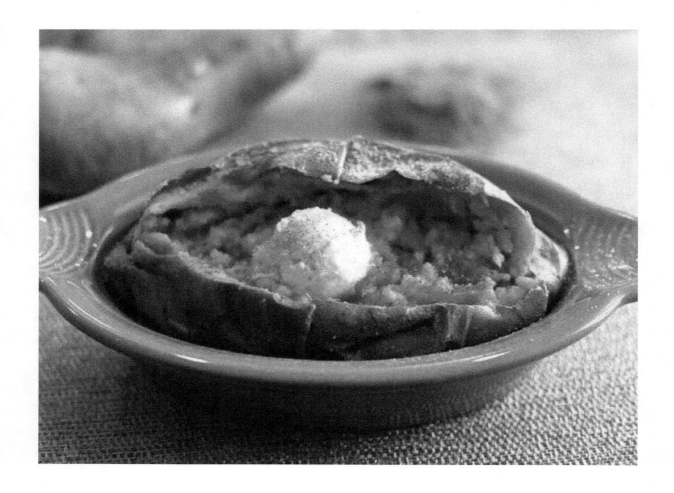

65. Lone Star Steakhouse & Saloon® Baked Sweet Potato

Preparation Time: 5 Minutes

Cooking Time: 25 Minutes

Servings: 8

Ingredients:

- 4 sweet potatoes
- Vegetable oil as required
- 3 tbsp. of sugar
- 1 ½ tsp. of ground cinnamon
- ½ cup of butter

Directions:

1. Preheat oven to 350°F.
2. Sprinkle some oil on the sweet potato skin and bake for 40–70 minutes, it depends on the size of the potatoes.
3. The outside will have dimmed when they are done and the inside is fuzzy.
4. You could see liquid from the sweet potato that is oozing when it's close to finish.
5. When baked with potatoes, combine sugar and cinnamon in small tub.
6. Slice one sweet potato down the center to serve.
7. Add 2 cubits of whipped butter and sprinkle.
8. Add sugar/cinnamon over top and serve!

Nutrition:

- Calories: 325 kcal
- Fat: 8g
- Carbs: 15g
- Protein: 1g

Chapter 5: Special Occasion Keto Recipes

66. Taquitos

Preparation Time: 15 Minutes

Cooking Time: 45 Minutes

Servings: 12

Ingredients:

- ½ an onion, diced
- 2 tbsps. of garlic paste (or minced garlic)
- 1 tsp of cumin
- 1 tsp of chili powder
- 2 cups of shredded chicken
- 2/3 cup of enchilada sauce (or any hot sauce of your preference)
- 4 tbsps. of tbsps. cilantro, chopped
- 2 cups of shredded cheddar cheese
- 2 cups of Monterey jack (or another cheese of your preference)
- ½ tbsp of mixed herb spice
- ½ cup of sour cream for serving
- 4 tbsps. of olive oil, divided

- Salt & pepper to taste

Directions:

1. Preheat the oven to 375ºF and line 2 baking trays with parchment paper.

2. Start by cooking the chicken if you haven't already; in a medium pan, heat up 2 tbsps. of oil over medium heat. Add in the onion, garlic paste and spices: cumin, chili powder, salt, and pepper. Stir for 1 minute until the onions have softened. Add in the chicken and shred it using 2 forks to pull the meat apart. Cook for about 5 minutes until the chicken is no longer pink. Add the cilantro into the pan and stir for another minute to mix all of the spices and ingredients together. Remove the pan from heat and set aside.

3. In a medium bowl, combine the 2 cheeses and mixed herb spice, then mix to combine. Evenly spread the cheese mix onto the baking trays, dividing it into 12 3" piles. Pop the trays into the oven and bake until the cheese has melted (about 10 minutes), keep an eye on the oven so that the cheeses don't burn. Remove the trays from the oven and allow the cheese shells to cool down.

4. Peel the cheese shells off of the parchment paper and spoon a generous amount of chicken into each cheese shell and then roll them tightly to secure the taquitos.

5. Serve with sour cream as a dip.

Nutrition:

- Calories: 230
- Carbohydrates:2 g
- Fat: 18 g
- Protein: 17 g

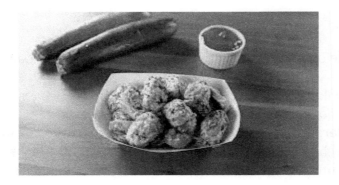

67. Zucchini Tater Tots

Preparation Time: 10 Minutes

Cooking Time: 30 Minutes

Servings: 4

Ingredients:

- 3 medium zucchinis, grated
- 2 eggs
- ½ cup of shredded cheddar cheese
- ½ cup of grated Parmesan
- 1 tsp of dried oregano
- ¼ tsp of cumin
- ¼ tsp of garlic powder

- Salt & pepper to taste
- ½ tsp of chili powder (optional, if you'd like a bit of spice)

Directions:

1. Preheat the oven to 400ºF and prepare a baking tray by lightly coating it with cooking spray.

2. Lay the grated zucchini onto a paper towel and pat it dry with another paper towel. Try to get it as dry as possible.

3. In a large bowl, crack the eggs and beat them with a fork/whisk until the liquid is light and fluffy. Add the grated zucchini in, along with the parmesan cheese, oregano, garlic powder, salt, cumin, chili powder (optional) and pepper. Mix the ingredients together until thick and well combined.

4. Using a tablespoon, spoon the mixture out and roll them into tiny balls, using your hands. Place the balls onto the baking sheet and bake the tater tots for about 15–20 minutes, turning the balls over, halfway through. Check for the golden, crisp texture to see if they're ready.

5. Serve with your favorite dipping sauce.

Nutrition:

- Calories: 220
- Carbohydrates: 7.3 g
- Fat: 12.8 g
- Protein: 21.9 g

68. Bell Pepper Nachos

Preparation Time: 15 Minutes

Cooking Time: 40 Minutes

Servings: 6

Ingredients:

- 4 bell peppers, washed, deseeded and shells cut into wedges (about the same size as nacho chips)
- 2 tbsps. of olive oil
- ½ tsp of cumin
- ½ tsp of chili powder
- ¼ tsp of garlic powder
- 1 ½ cups of shredded Monterrey Jack cheese
- 1 ½ cups of shredded cheddar cheese
- 1 cup of guacamole (recipe below for homemade guacamole)
- 1 cup of salsa (recipe below for homemade salsa)
- ½ cup of jalapenos, sliced
- ½ cup of sour cream
- 1 tbsp of milk
- ¼ cucumber, diced
- Salt & pepper to taste

- Lime wedges for serving

For homemade guacamole:

- 1 avocado
- ½ red onion, diced
- ½ tomato, diced
- A handful of cilantros
- A pinch of salt, pepper & cumin
- 1 tbsp of lime juice

For homemade salsa:

- 1 can of diced tomatoes
- 2 green chilis, chopped
- ½ an onion, diced
- 2 tbsps. of garlic paste
- 1 jalapeno, deseeded
- ½ tbsp of honey
- ½ cup of cilantro, chopped
- ½ lime's worth of juice
- Salt to taste

Directions:

1. Preheat the oven to 425ºF and line two baking trays with foil.

2. Prepare the guacamole by mashing the avocado into a smooth paste and mixing all of the ingredients into a bowl. Set aside.

3. Next, prepare the salsa by adding all of the ingredients (except the cilantro) into a blender. Blend until smooth. Add the cilantro in and set aside.

4. Lay the bell peppers on the baking sheet, hollow side facing up. Drizzle the bell pepper wedges with oil, then season with salt, pepper, cumin, chili powder and garlic powder. Pop the trays in the oven and bake for 10 minutes until the bell peppers are crisp on the outside and the flesh is tender.

5. Remove the trays and sprinkle the bell pepper wedges with the 2 cheeses. Pop the tray back in the oven for another 10 minutes until the cheese has melted.

6. While the cheese is melting, pour the sour cream, cucumber, and milk into a bowl. Sprinkle some pepper into the bowl and mix the contents together, then set aside.

7. Once the wedges are ready, top them with the guacamole, salsa and sliced jalapenos. Pour the sour cream mix over the top. Add a few lime wedges and enjoy!

Nutrition:

- Calories: 410

- Carbohydrates:13 g

- Fat: 32 g

- Protein: 17 g

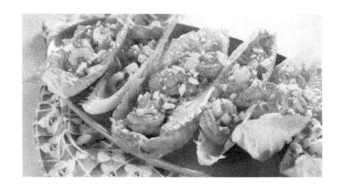

69. Buffalo Style Shrimp in Lettuce Wraps

Preparation Time: 15 Minutes

Cooking Time: 20 Minutes

Servings: 4

Ingredients:

- ¼ tbsp of butter
- 1 tbsp of garlic paste
- ¼ cup of hot sauce
- 1 tbsp of olive oil
- 1 lb. of shrimp, washed, peeled, deveined
- 1 head of romaine, washed and leaves separated
- ¼ red onion, chopped finely

- 1 rib of celery, thinly sliced
- ½ cup of crumbled blue cheese
- Salt & pepper to taste

Directions:

1. In a small pan over medium heat, add in the butter and stir until the butter has melted (about 2 minutes). Once the butter has melted, stir in the garlic paste and hot sauce, then lower the heat.

2. In a large pan over medium heat, pour in the shrimp and generously season with salt and pepper. Cook the shrimp for about 2 minutes on either side, until the shrimp is pink. Coat the shrimp in the butter sauce and turn the heat off. Stir the sauce to mix well with the shrimp.

3. Layer the lettuce leaves so that their hollow sides are facing upwards (to mimic a bowl). Spoon the shrimp into the hollow of each leaf, add a few slices of onion and celery, and sprinkle with blue cheese.

Nutrition:

- Calories: 263
- Carbohydrates: 8.7 g
- Fat: 11.5 g
- Protein: 31.6 g

70. Baby Back Ribs

Preparation Time: 5 Minutes

Cooking Time: 40 Minutes

Servings: 4

Ingredients:

- 2 lb. of baby back ribs
- ¼ cup of BBQ spice rub
- 2 tbsps. of apple cider vinegar
- ½ tsp of liquid smoke (this can be substituted for smoked paprika)
- BBQ sauce of your preference

Directions:

1. Clean the ribs thoroughly and then massage the spice rub into the ribs. Make sure to completely coat and massage the dry run into the meat, so that it's extra flavorful.

2. Pour 1 cup of water, vinegar and the liquid smoke into the pressure cooker and mix. Place the wire rack inside the pot, and then add the ribs onto the rack.

3. Lock the pressure cooker and set it to "sealed." Cook for 30 minutes on a medium-high.

4. Neutrally release the steam for about 5 minutes, then quick release. Set the oven to 400ºF and the function to "broil."

5. Place the ribs onto a baking tray and brush the ribs with the BBQ sauce of your choice. Pop the tray in the broiler for 5–7 minutes until the sauce has caramelized and thickened.

6. Alternatively, if you're at a BBQ, you can place the rack ribs on the grill for 10 minutes until the sauce has caramelized.

Nutrition:

- Calories: 451
- Carbohydrates: 24.1 g
- Fat: 24.3 g
- Protein: 25.5 g

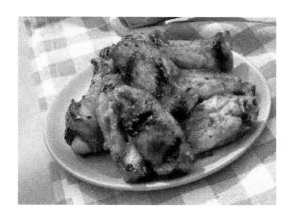

71. Grilled Buffalo Wings

Preparation Time: 10 Minutes

Cooking Time: 25 Minutes

Servings: 6

Ingredients:

- 4 lb. of chicken wings (about 30 wings)
- 3 cups of buttermilk
- 1 ¼ cups of buffalo sauce, divided (homemade recipe below)
- 1 tbsp of garlic powder
- 1 tbsp of dried oregano
- 1 tsp of cayenne pepper
- ½ tbsp of mixed herb spice

- ¼ cup of butter
- 1 tbsp of Worcestershire sauce
- 2 tbsps. of garlic paste
- Salt & pepper to taste

For the buffalo sauce:

- ½ cup of butter, melted
- ½ cup of hot sauce
- 2 tbsps. of white wine vinegar
- 2 tbsps. of Worcestershire sauce
- A pinch of garlic powder

Directions:

1. To prepare the buffalo sauce, melt the butter in a small bowl in the microwave for about 20 seconds.

2. In a medium bowl, mix the butter, hot sauce, vinegar, Worcestershire sauce and garlic powder. Stir well to combine. Place the sauce in a container and set aside.

3. To prepare the wings: in a large Ziplock back, add the wings, buttermilk and ¼ cup of the buffalo sauce in. Massage the wings with the sauce, through the plastic bag so that the marinade works its way into the meat. Place the plastic bag into a bowl and place in the refrigerator for 2 to 8 hours.

4. Once the wings have marinated, remove the wings from the marinade sauce, pat dry with a paper towel, then place the wings into a new, clean plastic bag.

5. Prepare a small bowl and pour in the garlic powder, oregano, mixed herb spice, salt, cayenne pepper and pepper. Pour the spice mixture into the plastic bag with the wings and once again, massage the spice mixture into the wings and leave to marinate at room temperature for 30 minutes.

6. Once the wings have marinated, preheat the oven to 450ºF and place the wings on a baking tray/grill and cook for 5–8 minutes. Rotate the wings and cook for another 8–10 minutes.

7. While the wings are cooking, mix 1 cup of buffalo sauce with butter, Worcestershire sauce, and garlic paste in a small pan over medium heat. Stir the ingredients for about 2 minutes until they're melted and mixed well. Remove from heat.

8. Once the wings are ready, add the wings into a large dish and pour the sauce from the pan over the wings. Mix well so the sauce covers the wings. Enjoy while it's hot!

Nutrition:

- Calories: 137
- Carbohydrates:1 g
- Fat: 10 g
- Protein: 9 g

72. Brie & Caramelized Onion Burgers

Preparation Time: 15 Minutes

Cooking Time: 45 Minutes

Servings: 6

Ingredients:

For the caramelized onions:

- 2 tbsps. of avocado oil
- 1 onion, sliced thinly
- ½ tsp of salt
- ¼ tsp of cinnamon

For the burger:

- 2 lb. of ground beef
- A pinch of salt
- A pinch of pepper
- 1 tsp of mixed herb spice
- ½ tsp of garlic powder
- 4 oz of Brie cheese

Directions:

1. For the caramelized onions, place a medium saucepan over medium-low heat and lightly drizzle some oil to coat the surface. Add the onion slices into the pan, along

with the salt and cinnamon. Cook slowly for 10–15 minutes, stirring regularly so that the onion slices soften.

2. Once the onions are done, prepare the burgers: in a large bowl, use your hands to mix together the beef, salt, pepper, mixed herbs and garlic powder. Then divide the mince into 6 equal parts.

3. Roll each part into a ball, using your hands, then flatten the ball into a patty. Divide each patty in half and place a dollop of Brie cheese and a few caramelized onions in the center of 1 of the halves. Top the patty off with the second half, so that the meat encompasses the Brie and onion filling.

4. Place the burger patties on a preheated grill, or in the oven at 400ºF for 5–6 minutes on either side. Alternatively, you can fry the burgers on a medium-high heat on a saucepan for 3–5 minutes on either side.

5. Serve with a salad of your choice.

Nutrition:

- Calories: 312

- Carbohydrates: 2.5 g

- Fat: 34.7 g

- Protein: 31 g

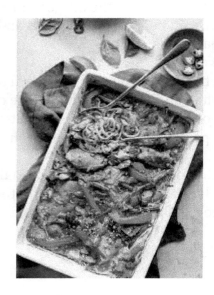

73. Chicken Zoodle Casserole

Preparation Time: 45 Minutes

Cooking Time: 45 Minutes

Servings: 4

Ingredients:

- 4 zucchinis
- ½ cup of Greek yogurt
- ½ cup of BBQ sauce (of your choice)
- 1 ½ cups of grated cheddar cheese, divided
- ½ tsp of paprika

- 1 cup of shredded chicken
- ½ cup of cilantro
- Salt & pepper to taste
- 1 tsp of garlic paste
- ½ tsp of turmeric
- ½ tsp of mixed herb spice
- 2 tbsps. of olive oil

Directions:

1. Preheat the oven to 200ºF and prepare 2 baking trays by lining them with paper towels.

2. Wash the zucchinis, then spiralize them using a blade (spiralize their thickness to your preference, but don't make them too thin or else they'll become crispy). Place the zucchini noodles onto the paper towels and season lightly with salt and paprika.

3. Pop the trays into the oven and bake the noodles for about 40 minutes, until they're dried out.

4. While the zucchini noodles cook, add the shredded chicken into a saucepan over medium heat. Add in the garlic paste, turmeric, salt, and pepper to taste. Drizzle the olive oil into the pan and fry the chicken for 2 minutes (if the chicken was already cooked) or 5 minutes (if uncooked), until the chicken is opaque and well coated in seasoning.

5. On another pan, prepare a medium-large skillet over medium-low heat, add in the Greek yogurt, BBQ sauce and 1 cup of the cheese. Cook the mixture for about 8–10 minutes, stirring slowly to melt and combine all of the ingredients. Set the cheese mixture and the shredded chicken aside. Once the zucchini noodles are ready, remove them from the oven and pat them dry with a paper towel. Raise the oven temperature to 375ºF.

6. In a medium bowl, add in the chicken, cilantro, mixed herb spice and zucchini noodles and gently mix together with a fork until well combined.

7. Pour the melted cheese sauce over the zucchini noodles and season once more with a sprinkle of pepper. Mix the ingredients well to evenly coat the noodles and chicken.

8. Prepare a casserole dish and pour the contents from the bowl into the casserole dish and place in the oven to bake for 20 minutes.

9. Remove the dish from the oven and set the option to broil. Sprinkle the remaining ½ cup of cheese over the top of the casserole dish and pop it back in the oven for another 10–15 minutes until the cheese is golden and crisp.

Nutrition:

- Calories: 285
- Carbohydrates: 21 g
- Fat: 10.2 g
- Protein: 24 g

74. Spicy Tuna Stuffed Avocados

Preparation Time: 10 Minutes

Cooking Time: 0 Minutes

Servings: 1

Ingredients:

- 1 avocado
- 1 small can of tuna
- ¼ red bell pepper, diced
- ¼ red onion, sliced thinly
- 1 tsp of mayonnaise
- 1 tsp of Dijon mustard
- 1 tsp of chives
- ½ of a lime's juice, divided
- Salt & pepper to taste
- Hot sauce for drizzling

Directions:

1. Halve the avocado and remove the pit.
2. Wash and prepare the vegetables: dice the pepper and slice the onion. Add it into a medium bowl.
3. Drain the canned tuna and add it into the bowl, along with the mayonnaise, Dijon mustard, salt, and pepper.

4. Chop up the chives and add it into the bowl, then mix it all together.

5. Spoon out the tuna, mix into the hollows of the avocados and squeeze more lime juice on top. Sprinkle a little extra pepper and drizzle with hot sauce of your choice.

Nutrition:

- Calories: 502
- Carbohydrates: 19 g
- Fat: 34 g
- Protein: 37 g

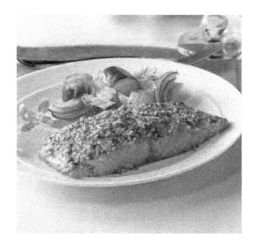

75. Pesto Salmon

Preparation Time: 5 Minutes

Cooking Time: 15 Minutes

Servings: 4

Ingredients:

- 1 lb. salmon fillet
- 2 tbsps. of olive oil/melted butter
- 20 cherry tomatoes
- ½ cup of dry white wine
- 1 tsp of rosemary
- 1 tsp of thyme

- Salt & pepper to taste
- 1 tsp of mixed herb spice
- 4 tsps. of sesame seeds
- ¼ cup of basil pesto
- Cauliflower rice/salad for serving (optional)

Directions:

1. Preheat the oven to 400ºF and prepare a baking tray by layering it with a sheet of foil.
2. Place the salmon onto the foil. Season the salmon with salt, pepper and mixed herb spice, then drizzle the oil/melted butter over the fish.
3. Pour the cherry tomatoes around the fish fillet and lightly season the tomatoes with pepper, rosemary and thyme. Fold the foil around the edges to create a rim of about 1" in height.
4. Pour the white wine into the foil pocket, generously coating the salmon and tomatoes.
5. Cover the fish and tomatoes with another layer of foil and press the edges of the foil to the bottom foil layer, tightly securing the contents inside.
6. Place the tray into the oven and cook for about 10 minutes, then remove the fish from the oven and keep it covered for another 5 minutes.
7. After about 5 minutes, remove the top layer of the foil and lightly brush the fish with the pesto.
8. Generously sprinkle the sesame seeds on top of the fish and serve warm.

Nutrition:

- Calories: 393
- Carbohydrates: 4 g

- Fat: 29 g
- Protein: 27 g

Chapter 6: Dessert Keto Recipes

76. Strawberry Shortcake (The Cheesecake Factory)

Preparation Time: 10 Minutes

Cooking Time: 25 Minutes

Servings: 6

Ingredients:

- 2/3 cup Swerve
- ¼ cup shortening
- 1 large egg
- 1 teaspoon vanilla extract
- ¼ teaspoon salt
- 1 ½ cups almond flour
- 2 teaspoons baking powder
- ½ cup almond milk
- 1 cup heavy whipping cream, whipped
- 1 ½ quart fresh or frozen strawberries, sliced

Directions:

1. Take a mixing bowl and add shortening and Swerve to this bowl.

2. Beat these ingredients together as you add vanilla and egg.

3. Mix salt, almond flour, and baking powder in another bowl. Add this dry mixture to the egg batter and mix well. Stir in almond milk and mix well until it makes a smooth batter.

4. Take a 9-inch square baking pan and grease it with cooking spray.

5. Add the shortcake batter to the baking pan and spread it evenly.

6. Set the oven's temperature to exactly 350ºF for preheating.

7. Place the shortcake pan in the oven for 25 minutes approximately.

8. Once baked, insert a toothpick into the shortcake to check if it is completely baked.

9. Place the hot baked cake on a wire rack and leave it for 10 minutes to cool it down.

10. Run a cake knife around the edges of the cake and remove it from the pan.

11. Remove the baked cake from its pan and slice it into nine equal-sized squares. Slice each square into half horizontally.

12. Add cream and strawberries in between the 2 layers of each cake square.

13. Make a sandwich with the 2 layers of the square and place them on the serving plates.

14. Garnish the shortcakes with desired toppings.

15. Serve.

Nutrition:

- Calories: 258
- Total Fat. 21.8 g
- Saturated Fat: 5.9 g
- Cholesterol: 58 mg

- Sodium: 139 mg
- Total Carbohydrates: 8.2 g
- Dietary Fiber: 3 g
- Total Sugars: 0.7 g
- Protein: 7.5 g

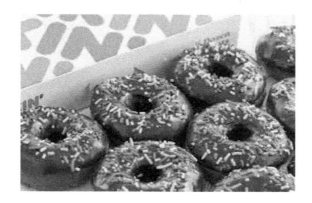

77. Chocolate Glazed Donuts (Dunkin Donuts)

Preparation Time: 10 Minutes

Cooking Time: 8 Minutes

Servings: 8

Ingredients:

- 2 ¼ cups almond flour
- 1 ¼ cups cocoa powder
- 2 teaspoons baking powder
- 1 teaspoon salt
- 4 large eggs
- 1 ½ cups granulated Swerve
- 5 tablespoons butter, softened

- 1/3 cup coconut milk
- 6 cups vegetable oil, for frying

Glaze:

- ½ cup almond milk
- 5 cups Swerve
- 2 teaspoons vanilla
- 1 pinch salt
- ½ cup sugar-free chocolate, melted

Directions:

1. Take a large bowl and add baking powder, salt, flour, and cocoa powder.
2. Mix these ingredients well and set this mixture aside.
3. Crack eggs into a steel mixing bowl and beat with an electric beater until the color changes to pale yellow.
4. Add coconut milk, butter, and Swerve; then beat again until smooth.
5. Now stir in flour mixture and continue mixing until it forms a smooth dough.
6. Transfer the prepared donut dough to a lightly floured surface and roll the dough so it is half an inch thick.
7. Cut 3-inch rounds out of this sheet, then cut ½-inch holes at the center of each round.
8. Place the donuts on a baking sheet, dusted with flour.
9. Set a steel cooling rack on a baking sheet and set it aside.
10. Prepare a deep pan and fill it with oil for deep frying.

11. Set the pan on medium-high heat and allow it to heat to 375ºF.

12. Now add donuts to the oil in batches and deep fry them for 2 minutes per side until golden-brown.

13. Once fried, remove the donuts from the oil and place them on a plate lined with a paper towel.

14. Mix everything for glaze in a saucepan and place it over medium heat.

15. Stir, cook this mixture for 4 minutes, then allow it to cool.

16. Dip the donuts in the chocolate mix.

17. Place the donuts in a serving tray and allow the chocolate glaze to set on top.

18. Serve fresh.

Nutrition:

- Calories: 356
- Total Fat: 0.6 g
- Saturated Fat: 7.5 g
- Cholesterol: 112 mg
- Sodium: 401 mg
- Total Carbohydrates: 1.5 g
- Dietary Fiber: 7.4 g
- Total Sugars: 1 g
- Protein: 12.5 g

78. Muffins (Dunkin Donuts)

Preparation Time: 10 Minutes

Cooking Time: 15 Minutes

Servings: 6

Ingredients:

- 1 cup almond flour
- 1 cup almond meal
- 3 tablespoons Swerve, granulated
- 1 tablespoon baking powder
- ½ teaspoon salt
- 2 eggs, beaten
- 1 cup of almond milk
- ½ stick butter, salted, melted, and cooled
- 2 tablespoons vegetable oil

Directions:

1. Set the oven's temperature at 425ºF for preheating.
2. Take a suitable muffin pan and grease it with butter, melted.
3. Place this muffin pan in the preheated oven until the muffin batter is completely ready.
4. Take a suitably-sized mixing bowl and add almond meal, flour, Swerve, baking powder, and salt.

5. Separately beat egg with oil, butter, melted, and milk in another bowl.

6. Make a small well at the center of the almond flour mixture and pour the egg mixture into this well.

7. Mix the dry flour mixture with the egg mixture and continue mixing until it forms a smooth batter.

8. Remove the muffin pan from the oven and place it on the working surface.

9. Pour an equal amount of batter into each muffin cup and allow it to set.

10. Transfer the prepared muffin tray to the oven and bake it for 15 minutes in the preheated oven.

11. Allow the well-baked muffins to cool at room temperature for 10 minutes.

12. Remove all the muffins from the tray and serve.

Nutrition:

- Calories: 390
- Total Fat: 35.4 g
- Saturated Fat: 15 g
- Cholesterol: 75 mg
- Sodium: 103 mg
- Total Carbohydrates: 11 g
- Dietary Fiber: 4.9 g
- Total Sugars: 2.1 g
- Protein: 11 g

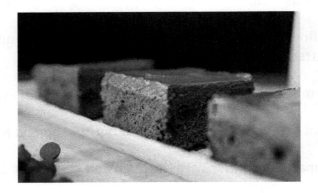

79. Frosted Fudge Brownies (Panera Bread)

Preparation Time: 10 Minutes

Cooking Time: 25 Minutes

Servings: 6

Ingredients:

- ½ cup and 1 tablespoon butter
- ¼ cup cocoa powder
- 2 large eggs
- 1 cup of Swerve
- ¾ cup almond flour
- ½ teaspoon baking powder
- ½ teaspoon salt

- ½ teaspoon vanilla extract

Frosting:

- 3 tablespoons butter, softened
- 1 1/3 cups Swerve
- ¼ cup baking cocoa
- ½ teaspoon vanilla extract
- 1/6 cup almond milk

Directions:

1. Take a suitable-sized saucepan and place it over medium heat. Add butter to this pan and let it melt over the heat.
2. Remove the buttered pan from the heat and stir in cocoa, then mix well. Keep this cocoa and butter mixture aside. Put eggs and Swerve in a large bowl, then stir well.
3. Stir in baking powder, salt, vanilla, melted cocoa mixture, and flour.
4. Mix these ingredients well until smooth and lump-free.
5. Take a 7-inch baking pan and grease it with cooking oil.
6. Spread the prepared cocoa butter in the pan.
7. Bake the fudge brownie batter for 25 minutes at 350ºF.
8. Once baked, insert a toothpick into the brownie to check if it is completely cooked.
9. Transfer the brownie pan to a wire rack and allow it to cool.
10. Meanwhile, whisk butter with Swerve in a mixing bowl for 7 minutes until fluffy and creamy.
11. Stir in vanilla and cocoa, then mix well. Add some milk if the glaze is too thick.

12.   Spread the glaze on top of the baked brownie. Slice and serve.

Nutrition:

- Calories: 125
- Total Fat: 8.8 g
- Saturated Fat: 1.3 g
- Cholesterol: 62 mg
- Sodium: 223 mg
- Total Carbohydrates: 5.3 g
- Dietary Fiber: 2.6 g
- Total Sugars: 0.2 g
- Protein: 5.8 g

80. Cinnamon Scones (Panera)

Preparation Time: 10 Minutes

Cooking Time: 30 Minutes

Servings: 8

Ingredients:

- 1 2/3 cups almond flour
- ¼ cup brown Swerve
- 2 teaspoons baking powder
- 1 teaspoon ground cinnamon
- 1/8 teaspoon salt
- 1 cup heavy whipping cream
- ½ cup sugar-free chocolate chips
- ½ cup pecans, toasted and chopped
- 1 tablespoon butter, melted

Glaze:

- ¼ cup Swerve
- 4 ½ teaspoons cream cheese
- 2 ¼ teaspoons almond milk
- ¼ teaspoon vanilla extract

Directions:

1. Take a large-sized bowl and add baking powder, brown Swerve, flour, salt, and cinnamon.
2. Whisk in cream, then mix until it all comes together into a dough.
3. Fold in pecans and chocolate chips.
4. Knead the dough 10 times on a lightly floured surface.
5. Place the pecan dough in a bowl and cover it with a plastic sheet.
6. Refrigerate the pecan dough for 30 minutes and allow it to set.
7. Spread this dough into 8-inch circles and cut it into 4–6 equal-sized wedges
8. Take a suitable-sized baking sheet and grease it with cooking oil or butter.
9. Spread the prepared dough wedges on the baking sheet.
10. Set the oven's temperature to 375ºF for preheating.
11. Once preheated, place the baking sheet in the oven and bake the scones for 30 minutes.
12. Meanwhile, prepare the glaze by mixing all its ingredients in a bowl.
13. When the scones are baked, remove them from the oven and place them on the wire racks.
14. Drizzle the cream cheese glaze over the baked scones and leave them for 10 minutes.
15. Serve fresh.

Nutrition:

- Calories: 213
- Total Fat: 18.7 g
- Saturated Fat: 5.3 g

- Cholesterol: 24 mg
- Sodium: 60 mg
- Total Carbohydrates: 6.4 g
- Dietary Fiber: 2.8 g
- Total Sugars: 0.1 g
- Protein: 5.4 g

Conclusion

Thank you for your support and finishing this book.

All of these recipes are beneficial for health-conscious people or obese people.

Carbohydrates should be taken according to the body's needs, but we usually ignore such facts and figures that would lead to incurable conditions. So, it is better not to take your metabolism and biological systems for granted and not take in higher proteins, carbohydrates, and fats.

Keto diet recipes are often healthy and meet your requirements to obtain your favorite foods with the same taste, color and flavor so that you can enjoy them thoroughly. You do not have to be self-conscious of your fat as it can be quickly burned by ketosis and give you another life. You need to monitor your diet regularly.

You have the freedom to eat anything like an average person, but with the required amount. Follow a diet plan that includes meat, eggs, vegetables, dairy products, and seafood.

Please don't run away from oil, as we are here to cut down on carbs, not fats. Carbohydrates, if not taken, would be harmful to the body, but it is better to refrain from them as it does not affect any organ, not even the brain, as it has been a myth for years that it harms the brain. Still, the keto diet stimulates bodily functions and prevents further absorption of carbohydrates into the bloodstream. The Keto Diet with keto copycat recipes will give you good health and give you another chance to be alive again.

Dieting does not have to mean deprivation. While the keto diet can be viewed as a restrictive diet, what it really is, is just a new way to approach what you eat. You don't have to dread never getting to enjoy a dessert or your favorite meals you loved ordering when you would go out to eat. You don't have to struggle to come up with exciting meals that will encourage you to stick to your goals.

The recipes in this book offer you with the first steps to learning how to cook the correct method while on the keto diet. You have been introduced to a number of new ingredients that allow you to still enjoy your favorite meals. These recipes can become your go-to for breakfast on the go and quick lunches, and even your kids will willingly sit down and eat dinner!

Now that you have everything you need to get started and have success on the keto diet, it is up to you to make the commitment and actually take the first step. I encourage you to start today! Create a meal plan that swaps out those unhealthy carbs and introduces more vegetables and lean meats. Choose one breakfast, lunch, and dinner recipe from this book to try this week. Don't be intimidated by the newness of this diet. Don't focus on what you will have to give up because, for the most part, there is almost always a keto-friendly alternative or copycat recipe that will make you realize this diet isn't as restrictive as you may have first believed.

Good luck!

CPSIA information can be obtained
at www.ICGtesting.com
Printed in the USA
LVHW100824250821
696050LV00004B/114